THE BOOK OF KOMBUCHA

THE BOOK OF KOMBUCHA

BETH ANN PETRO

ROBERT HOLMES

Photographer

Ulysses Press Berkeley, CA

1996

Published by: Ulysses Press
             P.O. Box 3440
             Berkeley, CA 94703-3440

Library of Congress Catalog Card Number: 95-61972

ISBN: 1-56975-049-1

Printed in the USA by R R. Donnelley & Sons

10 9 8 7 6 5 4 3 2 1

Editorial and production: Leslie Henriques, Joanna Pearlman, Lee Micheaux,
    Claire Chun, Jennifer Wilkoff
Cover Design: Sarah Levin
Front cover photograph: P. Amranand/SuperStock
Indexer: Sayre Van Young
Kitchen courtesy of Scott Cameron

Distributed in the United States by Publishers Group West, in Canada by Raincoast Books, and in Great Britain and Europe by World Leisure Marketing.

TABLE OF CONTENTS

ACKNOWLEGMENTS

There is no way that this book could have been written without the research and moral support from my business partner and sister, Gayle Skowronski. Susan Prather also deserves credit for steering me onto the "information superhighway," helping me find my way through computer on-line research databases and the internet. And thanks to everyone who shared their kombucha stories with me.

INTRODUCTION

Kombucha. Ask strangers on the street if they've heard of it and they will likely stop to think for a moment, then smile and reply, "Yes. Isn't it some sort of mushroom that you can make a tea out of?"

You can hear talk of kombucha everywhere—on TV, from your hair stylist, on the internet. I even overheard a florist discussing kombucha while she was preparing my wedding bouquet. You may hear kombucha praised as the miracle cure for any ill. You may hear it condemned as the latest quackery. As you will see when you read this book, the truth is somewhere in between.

So, should you try experimenting with this magic mushroom? Brewing and drinking the kombucha beverage can be fun and educational. It may make you feel better and more energetic. Unless you already have a serious health problem, it's not likely to cause you harm. However, you need to make your own decision about using kombucha. This book will give you as complete and accurate information as possible about kombucha. You'll learn what kombucha is and how it works, according to the most recent research. The book also relates the many folklore accounts of where kombucha came from and describes the benefits many have experienced from using it. I'll also share step-by-step instructions for how to make and use the kombucha brew and answer common questions about kombucha. The book does not endorse or prescribe the kombucha brew for curing specific health problems. Read on to learn more about this exotic substance and its brew. Then form your own opinion. Whatever you decide about kombucha, you'll be more knowledgeable about your health and the amazing life processes of the world around you.

1

WHAT IS KOMBUCHA?

"...A blob-like white fungus . . ."
> —London Times

"...that clones itself . . ."
> —New York Times

"...has spread like a New Age chain letter . . ."
> —Palm Beach Post

"...like the inexorable spread of bathroom mildew . . ."
> —American Medical News

"...has an intelligence well above the level of a dolphin . . ."
> —Norman Baker in the Chicago Tribune

Bathroom mildew? Greater intelligence than a dolphin? Just what is this kombucha mushroom thing that causes people to spin off such colorful phrases? To find out, you'll need to take a closer look at a bowl of kombucha culture and its tea.

The kombucha (pronounced kum-BOO-sha) culture is beige and somewhat opaque. The official pharmaceutical name for the culture is *Fungus japonicus*. Kombucha usually is shaped like a large pancake. That's because it grows to conform to the shape of the container it's in. The exception to this is if you purchase a culture from the largest distributor of the kombucha culture in the U.S., Laurel Farms. Then your culture arrives cut into a cute little heart shape.

Over time, the kombucha culture thickens to just under half an inch, unless you're like me and live in a cooler area like the central California coast. In that case, the culture may stay thinner—mine stays at about a quarter of an inch thick. The "mother" culture, purchased from Laurel Farms (coming from the warmer southern part of the state), was twice as thick. The thickness may vary somewhat with the seasons, thicker in the summer and thinner in the winter. Besides thickening up, the culture gradually creates new "pancakes" that usually rest on top of the old ones.

If you pick up the kombucha culture, you'll find it to be slippery and flexible. It could even be described as somewhat slimy. When it's young, it's fairly fragile. As it ages, the kombucha is more durable,

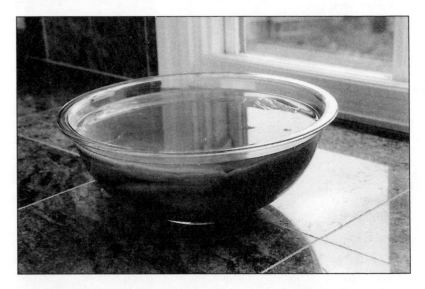

The beige kombucha culture usually floats on a bath of black tea.

feels tougher and is easier to handle. Generally, the culture floats on top of tea. However, it may occasionally decide to rest at the bottom.

Kombucha has been referred to as a sponge, lichen, mold, algae, seaweed and who knows what else. Besides these and other, more fanciful names, kombucha is most typically referred to as a mushroom. However, one of the first things you'll hear from anyone who wants to flaunt his or her knowledge about kombucha is the emphatic statement that kombucha is *not* a mushroom. In fact, that jellyfish-like object floating on a bowl of black tea is not a single organism at all. Actually, the kombucha culture's main components is best described as a friendly meeting of yeasts and bacteria, encased in cellulose.

Yeast

Yeast is considered a type of fungus, along with molds and mushrooms and various other strange, somewhat slimy organisms. First, let's take a look at some of the basic characteristics of the fungus family. Unlike your green leafy plants, fungi don't have the ability to create their own food. They must find their food from organic matter—from carbohydrates (sugars) in particular—whether the matter is decaying, starting to die or even still living. That's why you'll find mushrooms growing wherever there are lots of old leaves rotting on the ground, molds growing on old bread and maybe even (ugh!) a telltale red rash on your foot from the fungus that causes athlete's foot. But what does that have to do with yeast and kombucha?

Yeasts are simple fungal creatures much smaller than mushrooms—in fact, they're only one cell in size. If you carried a microscope around with you, you'd see yeasts everywhere: on leaves and skin, in soil and water and even inside your intestinal tract. They're found just about anywhere you find carbohydrates. And the more of these sugars the yeasts eat, the quicker the yeasts reproduce.

Fungi—and yeasts—reproduce in a few ways: 1) by scattering spores (mushrooms and the candida yeast are two good examples of this), 2) by splitting (similar to cell division in bacteria) and 3) by "budding."

This last method of reproduction is the one preferred by the kombucha yeasts.

Three types of beneficial bacteria reside in the kombucha culture.

The yeasts and the byproducts yeasts give off when eating and reproducing have been "harnessed" for a variety of useful purposes: Yeasts give off carbon dioxide to make bread rise. Yeasts have been used to create powerful medications to treat many types of illnesses, including infections and cancer. Yeasts have also been used in practically every society to ferment grains and fruits. The results? Well-preserved alcoholic beverages ranging from beer (usually made from barley) to sake (made from rice).

Yeasts also contain substances that are beneficial to you. These include minerals, vitamins, proteins, and substances called "sterols." Sterols are chemicals found in the cell walls of every living organism. They're sort of waxy, don't easily dissolve in water, and serve many different purposes. The sterol you're probably most familiar with is cholesterol, which not only can clog up your arteries but also lines your nerves, serves as the protective coat on your skin, and provides many other helpful benefits. Ergosterol is the primary sterol found in yeast cells. It's also another sterol that your body finds a use for. When exposed to sunlight, ergosterol changes into Vitamin D, which helps your bones use calcium.

Bacteria

Bacteria reside with yeasts in the kombucha culture. Also single-celled organisms, bacteria may have been the first life form on earth. They're stubborn survivors, found even in frozen soil, hot water, the upper atmosphere and the deep ocean. In the biological "pecking order," bacteria fall somewhere between plants and yeasts. Like yeasts, most bacteria can't grow their own food and must rely on other plant and animal sources. Bacteria need something to help them break down this food into energy. One type of bacteria uses oxygen to generate energy: aerobic (living with oxygen) bacteria. Another type of bacteria uses substances other than oxygen, such as enzymes, nitrogen or sulfur, to generate energy. They are called anaerobic (living without oxygen) bacteria.

Many bacteria create cellulose as one of the byproducts of digestion. However, the bacteria cell walls are made up not of cellulose but of murein, a combination of sugars and acids. This use of murein rather than cellulose in bacterial cell walls explains why penicillin kills bacteria without hurting you. Penicillin prevents the formation of murein. Luckily, your cell walls are made of cellulose instead.

Bacteria come in a variety of shapes: rods, spheres and spirals. Under ideal conditions, they can reproduce rapidly—from one bacterium to over 500,000 bacteria in less time than it takes you to complete a typical work day—about six hours.

We generally think of bacteria as "bad," the cause of many human diseases. After all, such potentially serious problems as food poisoning and strep throat are caused by bacteria. But most bacteria are harmless, beneficial or even essential to our existence. Every time you nibble on a wedge of cheese, eat a quick lunch of yogurt, or sprinkle vinegar on your salad, you're benefiting from the work done by bacteria. Bacteria change that compost pile of grass clippings in the corner of your back yard into rich humus for your garden. Bacteria are used to break down raw sewage at your local water treatment plant. And, you'll find bacteria at work in kombucha.

In the kombucha brew, bacteria finish the work begun by the yeasts, eating alcohol and leaving behind acids. The process is similar to making vinegar, except that commercial vinegar production doesn't use yeast. Rather, it starts further along the process with alcohol (wine or hard cider) and introduces bacteria into the liquid. However, the end results are similar. In fact, the French roots of the word "vinegar" describe the kombucha brew's taste rather accurately: *vin* (wine) and *aigre* (sour). More about that later.

Cellulose

Kombucha wears a tough coat of cellulose, which protects the yeasts and bacteria.

Cellulose is actually a very complex carbohydrate, or sugar. It's fibrous and doesn't dissolve in water, making it an ideal structure for many living organisms, most notably for plants and even for your body's own cells. You can find cellulose all around you: in flowers and trees, in natural fabric fibers such as cotton, flax and ramie, and in industrial products such as cellophane, film and rayon. You'll also find cellulose in the kombucha culture.

No one is certain why the cellulose is created by the bacteria. It is assumed that the cellulose evolved as a dwelling for both the bacteria and the yeasts. It may also keep the bacteria close to oxygen, as well as protect them from light. You'll recognize the cellulose as the tough outer coating of the kombucha culture.

The Three-In-One Culture Meets Tea

Yeast, bacteria, and cellulose—the three main components of the kombucha culture. Now you know a little bit more about all three. But this knowledge has probably generated even more questions. Where did this strange culture come from? How does it produce the kombucha beverage? What does tea have to do with it? Which yeasts and bacteria are in the kombucha culture? Are any of them harmful to people? So many questions. Read on to find out more about the history of the kombucha culture and how it continues to survive and thrive.

2

WHERE DID KOMBUCHA COME FROM?

The kombucha culture is quite a world traveler. If you know where to look and what to call it, you can find the culture and its brew in China, Japan, India, Korea, Java, the Philippines, Russia, Eastern Europe, Germany, the United Kingdom, the United States, Canada and Brazil. Apparently it was even a big hit in South Africa in the early 1990s.

How the culture was originally conceived and how it spread to all these places is not really known. But the stories that have come to be associated with kombucha's creation and history are fascinating—even though they may be completely impossible to verify. At the very least, the lore surrounding kombucha makes for interesting reading. The various tales about kombucha's spread and its numerous names show just how interested people throughout the world have been in this strange and amazing substance.

One fact is clear. The kombucha culture has its origins somewhere in the East, perhaps China, Korea, Russia or India. Most likely it was "discovered" in China, and then moved south to Korea, southwest to India and north to Russia.

It's probably safe to say that the culture wasn't found lying on some soft, peat-lined forest floor. Rather, it was probably concocted—deliberately or mistakenly—by someone who either knew something about fermentation or who was experienced in using fungi, yeast or bacteria cultures to brew beverages for medicine or enjoyment. In either case, after the serendipitous discovery of kombucha, the culture spread like wildfire. Or at least that's how it seems, viewing it from our perspective a few thousand years later.

Let's take a closer look at some of the lore associated with kombucha. I'll start in the East, where the culture is most likely to have originated.

Manchuria and China

In many ways, it only makes sense that devising, brewing and drinking the kombucha culture beverage would have originated somewhere in China. After all, the medium of the kombucha beverage itself—that is, tea—had its start in China, probably in the area where China, India and Myanmar (formerly called Burma) join together.

According to one story explaining the discovery of tea, the beverage was first used medicinally more than 4000 years ago, long before it became the socially acceptable drink of choice throughout Asia. It goes something like this: A Chinese emperor was boiling a pot of water, when a tea leaf fell into the pot. He tasted it and determined that it made pretty good medicine.

It's likely that the kombucha culture was developed much the same way, but this time in Manchuria in the far northeastern region of China, possibly as long ago as 220 B.C., during the Tsin dynasty. Regardless of its exact origins, the kombucha tea's popularity and reputation grew. The Chinese had already developed a healthy respect for the power of fungi, seeing them as magical and as a means of attaining immortality.

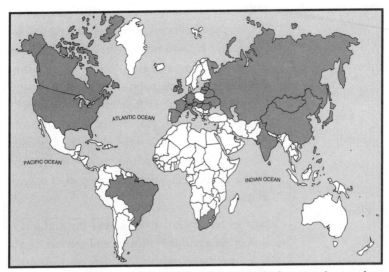

Kombucha has developed an active travel log over the last two thousand years (shaded areas indicate evidence of kombucha's use).

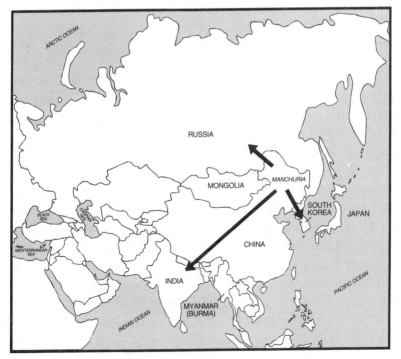

It's likely that kombucha originated in Asia, probably in Manchuria.

The origin of tea occurred 2000 years before kombucha, probably in the mountainous region where China, India and Myanmar meet.

"Divine Tea" *(Ling-tche)* was the name of one kombucha-like fungus that was already in use in Southern China to treat gastrointestinal distress. Kombucha became simply one more fungus with revered medicinal properties. By calling the kombucha brew the "Remedy for Immortality," it appears that the Manchurians took the kombucha beverage quite seriously. In fact, residents supposedly still drink the brew from the kombucha culture every morning as part of religious atonement.

Just as tea spread from China throughout the rest of Asia and into Europe and the West, so has the kombucha culture and beverage found its way from China to many countries throughout the world.

Korea, Japan and the Rest of Asia

Japan was probably one of the first areas outside of China where people began brewing and using the kombucha culture. If you look at a globe, you can see how easy it would have been for the kombucha culture to head south from Manchuria to Korea to Japan. Exactly how this happened isn't entirely clear but folklore suggests that a Korean physician, Dr. Kombu, was called to Japan over 1500 years ago—in about 415 A.D.—to treat the Emperor Inkyo for some sort of digestive disorder. Apparently the good Dr. Kombu used the kombucha brew as part of the emperor's therapy. It must have been effective, because the kombucha beverage became a bit hit. In fact, it looks like we get the name for this culture from this early Japanese encounter. Another version of the story states that the word "kombucha" is a combination of the Korean doctor's family name, "Kombu," and the Japanese word for "tea," *cha*. Change the "k" to "c" and you'll get the Japanese word for the culture, *combucha*. Others assert that the word comes from the

Japanese term for "seaweed," *kombu*. According to this version of the naming of kombucha, the Japanese either originally brewed the culture in a seaweed-based tea or mistook the culture itself for a type of seaweed. Still another explanation for the kombucha name suggests that it is derived from the Japanese word for "divine," *kambou*. Kombucha has also been called *kouchakinoko*, the black tea mushroom.

However the culture got its name, the kombucha beverage's use was apparently widespread in Japan, even to the point of warriors carrying it with them in flasks into battle. When the beverage's supply ran low, they simply filled up the flask with fresh tea, allowing the culture to continue to ferment. And even though its use slowly decreased in later times, kombucha has apparently been resurrected in the past 20 years as a healthy and refreshing beverage.

There are also reports of the kombucha culture's use throughout the rest of Asia, including Java, the Philippines and India. Look up some old copies of the *Tea Quarterly* published in Sri Lanka, and you'll find occasional references to the kombucha brew, often called "tea cider" in the publication.

Russia, the Former Soviet Union and Eastern Europe

Nobody is really sure when or how kombucha found its way into Russia. But take another look at the map. You'll note right away on the far eastern side of Asia that there's a shared border between the mountainous areas of the former Soviet Union and the so-called birthplace of kombucha, Manchuria. It's likely that traders coming from the south brought the kombucha culture along with other goods and introduced the brewing technique to their northern neighbors. In any case, however it arrived there, kombucha has apparently been part of life in small Russian mountain communities for a long time.

In Russia, the most common term for the kombucha beverage is "tea kvass," *cainii kvass*. Kvass itself is a weak Russian beer brewed from

"Kargasok tea," named after a small mountain village where kombucha has been used for years, is the term often used in Russia to describe kombucha brew.

bread, using a process that is similar to kombucha brewing. Instead of a yeast-fungal culture, kvass uses bread and baking yeast. The brewing medium is water, rather than tea. In addition to sugar, kvass also contains raisins. The resulting beverage contains only a low level of alcohol. I haven't seen a specific alcohol content listed for kvass, but it's probably similar to or less than that of the kombucha beverage, around 0.5 percent, which doesn't even qualify it as "lite" beer. Besides drinking kvass, you can also use it as a stock for soups such as borscht. (If you're interested in brewing kvass yourself, you can probably find a recipe in a Russian or Ukranian cookbook at your local library.) Perhaps it's the similarities between kvass and kombucha in brewing and taste that made kombucha so easily and widely accepted throughout Russia and Eastern Europe.

Another term used frequently to describe the kombucha brew in Russia and sometimes heard in the United States is "Kargasok tea." This phrase has been found on brewing instructions from an unknown author. The name apparently came about when a Japanese woman traveling through Russia visited Kargasok. She noted that brewing and drinking the kombucha beverage was apparently part of each family's daily routine.

It appears that the use of the kombucha culture was limited to Kargasok and other small mountain Russian villages for many years. However, some people in the Russian scientific community were aware of it early on. If you're persistent, you can find articles as far back as the 1910s and 1920s describing kombucha and its benefits.

But apparently the Soviet leader Joseph Stalin is the one to thank for popularizing kombucha throughout Eastern Europe. As the story goes, kombucha became more widespread in the Soviet Union as a result of Stalin's fear of cancer. Whether for personal reasons or simply for the good of the country, Stalin sent out Soviet cancer researchers to determine why cancer had become such a problem in so many areas of the

Soviet Union. It's said that the researchers conducted an exhaustive epidemiological study using the tactics of—and even perhaps with the help of—the KGB (the Soviet intelligence and internal security agency). They found two small areas with extremely low cancer rates, despite heavy environmental damage due to mining and factory operations. Lifestyle and other factors were closely analyzed, revealing nothing out of the ordinary. Finally, one of the lead researchers visited a family and was offered a refreshing beverage that turned out to be "tea kvass"— kombucha tea. The researchers determined that the beverage was used throughout the two communities. They also found that in spite of heavy pollution and extreme use of alcohol and tobacco, residents had low rates of cancer, low rates of alcoholism and high work productivity.

Apparently the results were impressive enough that Stalin himself was prescribed the kombucha brew by his personal physician. However, this led to one of Stalin's notorious purges. This particular purge of the Kremlin medical staff was well-reported, although it wasn't linked to kombucha until after the fact. Two KGB generals looking for yet another promotion claimed that Stalin's doctor was poisoning him with the kombucha beverage, resulting in the doctor's imprisonment. These generals published stories linking kombucha use to cancer. It's no surprise that drinking the brew then fell in popularity. But after Stalin's sudden and unexplained death in 1953, the tables turned. The generals ended up in prison and were later executed. Stalin's physician was released from prison and vindicated. Kombucha use rose in popularity once again. For the next few decades, scientific articles about kombucha in the Soviet Union and other Eastern European countries flourished. In the U.S.S.R., kombucha experiments were conducted in prisons and labor camps. Apparently, even the famed Russian writer Aleksandr Solzhenitsyn was treated with kombucha—or something very similar—as a cure for cancer. In his novel *Cancer Ward*, Solzhenitsyn describes a cancer therapy used in an area just outside of Moscow. The character Oleg Kostoglotov tells his desperate fellow patients of a letter he received from a physician who discovered that the peasants in the area he was serving had no cancer. The doctor attributed this to a tea the peasants drank, which was made from a fungus found on birch trees.

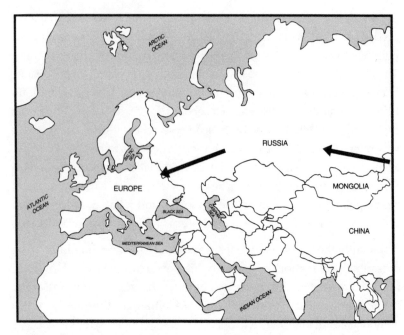

Kombucha traveled north through mountainous terrain into eastern Russia and then into Europe.

As the kombucha brew spread throughout Russia and Eastern Europe, other names for the culture and its resulting beverage arose. The culture is sometimes called *brinum-ssene* in Latvia, *cainii grib* in Russia, *cainogo griba* in Georgia, *chamboucho* in Romania and *olinka* in Bohemia and Moravia (regions within the current Czech and Slovenian Republics). The brew from the kombucha culture has several names as well, including *teyi saki* (Armenia) and *cainogo kvassa* (Georgia).

Germany and the Rest of Europe

Red tea, tea cider, Volga fungus, Russian jelly fish—the names Europeans have given to the kombucha culture and brew are colorful and numerous. In France, you'll hear the kombucha brew called *champignon de longue vie* (long-life mushroom). *Funko cinese* (Chinese fungus) is what the culture is known as in Italy. It's *hongo* in Spain. The Hungarians call it *Japán gomba*. And the Dutch phrase for the culture is *theezwam komboecha*.

How did kombucha reach Europe? There are two differing accounts, both tracing the path of kombucha from Russia to Germany. Some folks report that Russian sailors brought kombucha to Germany sometime in the 1800s. Another story is that Russian and German prisoners of war brought the culture to Germany. Both accounts may be true. In any case, it seems that by the end of the 1800s and through World War II, medical doctors and researchers in Germany studied the culture and brew quite extensively.

However it arrived in Germany, the kombucha culture (called *Teepilz*—tea mushroom) gradually earned the respect of various health care professionals, who recommended the brew for a variety of ills. There were several articles published from the early 1900s up until World War II that extolled the virtues of the beverage *Kombuchagetränk* ("kombucha drink"). However, kombucha brewing halted during World War II, probably because both tea and sugar became scarce throughout Europe. After the war, as the primary brewing ingredients became available once again, kombucha brewing spread to the rest of Europe.

Perhaps the strongest advocate of kombucha was the German physician Rudolf Sklenar. For 36 years after World War II and until his death in 1987, Sklenar, a medical doctor, prescribed the beverage and an extract from the kombucha culture itself as therapy for many patients with intestinal problems and chronic illnesses such as cancer. He called using these somewhat unorthodox treatments "outsiders' methods," knowing full well that he risked becoming the laughingstock of the medical community. His niece, Rosina Fasching, documents Sklenar's use of kombucha in her book, *Tea Fungus Kombucha: The Natural Remedy and Its Significance in Cases of Cancer and Other Metabolic Diseases*. Unfortunately, neither Sklenar nor Fasching made any attempt to document kombucha's effectiveness in a controlled scientific environment. And many view Sklenar as "a little off anyway," since he advocated unusual views about cancer.

Sklenar was convinced that cancer was simply a chronic metabolic disorder and that the cancerous growth itself was merely a symptom of another underlying problem. He believed that using radiation or chemotherapy to kill cells indiscriminately was only a short-term solution that often did more damage—to healthy cells—than good. He thought that any treatment of cancer or similar diseases had to start with correcting the off-balance metabolism, which itself was probably due to an underlying biological imbalance. Remedying the biologic imbalance could be accomplished by prescribing certain compounds—such as the kombucha extract and beverage—that contained beneficial bacteria, yeasts and other substances. These substances could suppress the action of the harmful bacteria thus restoring digestion and proper metabolism. The cancer would be stabilized and might even recede.

Sklenar didn't go so far as to say his methods "cured" cancer. Rather, he was hopeful that a vaccine would be developed to prevent cancer. He advocated that his treatment regimen would prolong life, alleviate side effects and eliminate many complications associated with cancer. Sklenar also believed that cancer was caused by the same virus, HIV, that leads to AIDS. But what really put Sklenar over the edge in the eyes of the academic medical community was his belief that cancer and other diseases could be diagnosed by examining a person's irises, the ringlike areas of color in the eyes.

No matter what you think about Sklenar's theories, we have one main accomplishment to thank him for. His years of experience with the kombucha culture led him to establish the standard kombucha brewing recipe, which is recommended—with only slight variations—by every credible resource you'll encounter. It is interesting to note, however, that Sklenar's niece *now* recommends that you not brew the culture yourself. She is suspicious of the many cultures and brewing instructions that have been used since the recent rebirth of kombucha in southern Germany and Austria. She thinks that many of these cultures aren't even kombucha cultures. Of course, Fasching may have a somewhat vested interest in commercially prepared kombucha beverage and extracts—the Dr. Sklenar® brands are exported and sold throughout the world.

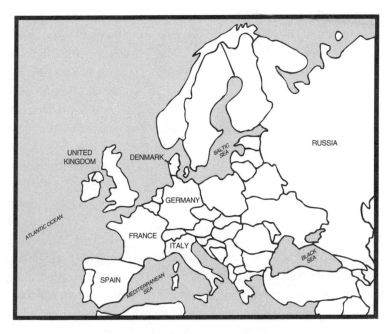

Kombucha arrived in Europe via Germany, probably in the late 1800s.

But back to the rest of Europe: The kombucha culture doesn't reside only in Germany. It has found its way to the rest of Europe, as well, though its popularity has been somewhat cyclical. One account states that the kombucha beverage was popular in Italy in the 1950s until rumors began circulating—most likely the very same rumors created by the KGB in the Soviet Union—that it caused cancer. These rumors are ironic since many of the components of the kombucha brew (such as vitamin C) have been linked to cancer prevention and amelioration of cancer symptoms.

However, use of the kombucha culture in Europe has been growing for the last decade or so. In addition to its continued presence in Italy, you can purchase the kombucha culture in many pharmacies in Switzerland, where it's called *Mo-Gu*. It's also found in France, the Netherlands, Hungary and Spain.

One reason the kombucha culture is so popular in Europe is the tireless advocacy of Günther Frank, a German who has spent years studying the culture, its history and its uses. Frank's qualifications are simply that he is interested in the beverage. He is neither scientist nor physician. But he's a potent spokesperson for kombucha. Besides making a strong case for kombucha's use in Europe, Frank is probably the person most responsible for sending kombucha across the Atlantic to the United States, by selling his books and the kombucha culture and being readily available to answer questions and exchange information.

North America

In the United States, the popularity of the kombucha culture and its beverage is a relatively young phenomenon. You'll hear it called many things in the U.S., among them the Manchurian mushroom and kombucha tea (a phrase that Laurel Farms is attempting to trademark, which is why in this book I usually refer to the tea as the brew or the beverage).

Kombucha has probably been around in the United States as long as there have been immigrants from Asia and Russia. Many children of immigrants from these regions vaguely recall their grandparents or parents brewing a sour-smelling substance in a pot kept in an inconspicuous corner. That substance was probably the kombucha beverage. However, the kombucha culture's popularity was limited until the early 1990s. *Search for Health* magazine was probably first to actively promote the kombucha culture. They learned about the beverage from a reader suffering from multiple sclerosis (MS) who started drinking the kombucha brew in 1989, with effective results. Since they had a clear focus on studying the health benefits of fermented products, they were eager to investigate the report further. Their search for information led them to the two main "western" works on the subject: books by Frank and Fasching. *Search for Health* and its parent company, Valentine Communications, has become the U.S. distributor of these books and continues to publish articles on kombucha and other similar kinds of substances.

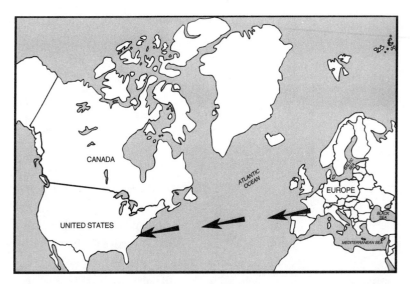

The big interest in kombucha in North America (Canada and the United States) started in the early 1990s.

But it's one woman's determination to find a way to fight AIDS and other chronic diseases that has really triggered the kombucha explosion in the United States. Betsy Pryor heard about the beverage in 1993 from her meditation teacher, who brought it back from a visit to China. Some souvenir! Pryor tried the beverage and felt immediate benefits, including more energy and clearer skin. She heard of others having even more dramatic health benefits. Pryor wondered if perhaps providing kombucha cultures was the answer to her search for ways to help people with AIDS and other chronic illness. In early 1994, Pryor and her partner, Norman Baker, started their own "kombucha farm." Thus began Laurel Farms, which in a short time has become the largest and most reliable U.S. grower and distributor of kombucha cultures. Ms. Pryor has furthered the cause of kombucha by appearing on numerous television and radio talk shows. Remaining true to her original goal, kombucha cultures are distributed by Laurel Farms at cost to people with AIDS and other chronic illnesses.

> *It is now estimated that at least three million Americans are brewing and drinking kombucha.*

And now it is estimated that three million Americans or more are brewing and drinking the beverage. This includes those with celebrity status as well as millions of everyday folks like you and me. Leeza Gibbons, a television personality, is trying out the kombucha beverage as part of her "healthy selfishness" plan to maintain her health in the face of a tightly packed life. She was skeptical at first, as can be witnessed on one segment of her talk show devoted to the topic. But Leeza justifies her health plan like this: "I meet people every day who are struggling with some sort of health problem. It's a reminder to protect what you have." The producer of her show informed me that the segment was so popular and they've received so many calls, that their entire staff has memorized the Laurel Farms address and phone number.

Word has it that even President Ronald Reagan drank the kombucha beverage after cancerous polyps were removed from his colon. He apparently received information about the culture and its beverage from Aleksandr Solzhenitsyn, and located a culture in Japan.

Because of the surging interest in the kombucha culture and beverage, U.S. researchers are also beginning to investigate the substance. Cornell University, Mt. Sinai School of Medicine and even the FDA are just a few of the organizations conducting research into kombucha. The insatiable search by Americans for that ever-elusive "fountain of youth" is being felt, even in the halls of academia.

And the Rest of the World

We've already mentioned that there was a "kombucha craze" in South Africa in the early 1990s. Kombucha has been found elsewhere, too. One kombucha-culture article with no ascribed author circulates in Brazil. It not only provides instructions for brewing the beverage, but also gives plenty of advice—some of it a little odd—on using the beverage for purposes beyond drinking. It also calls the culture "marine algae."

Are You Included in Kombucha's Itinerary?

So kombucha has found its way into the kitchens of people living in countries throughout the world. Whether brought by ancient traders crossing mountainous terrain or shipped in plastic baggies through Priority Mail, this fascinating culture certainly gets around. But how do you get one for your very own? Call the kombucha hotline? Take a trip to Manchuria? You'll be happy to know that, if you're interested, you can probably find a source for kombucha quite close to home.

3

FEED KOMBUCHA
AND WATCH IT GROW

"The mushrooms are living organisms and like to be touched."
—Comment from the America Online
Kombucha Message Board

It's true that the kombucha culture is a living, growing organism that has found its way around the world. Whether it grows better when fondled is an experiment you can consider undertaking. I, frankly, try to minimize contact with my kombuchas, so there's less risk of contamination to the culture. In any case, once the kombucha culture is placed in sweetened black tea, an almost magical process begins.

Remember the three main components of the kombucha culture we discussed in Chapter 1: yeast, bacteria and cellulose? Just sitting there by themselves, they'll starve and become a mushy, stinky mass not fit to reside in your Pyrex bowl. But give them some nourishment, and they go on a feeding frenzy. The process is rather complex. And it's not completely understood by anybody. But take a deep breath and pay attention. Soon you'll get the general idea of how the kombucha culture grows in tea.

For the kombucha process to occur, you need both a kombucha culture and something liquid for it to grow in (sometimes called a "medium"). The most commonly used liquid is black tea sweetened with plain old white sugar. Black tea contains substances that aid the brewing process: caffeine, oxygen, nitrogen, tannic acid, vitamins and some minerals. The sugar in the tea is a simple carbohydrate that provides nutrition for the yeasts and bacteria.

> *Plain old white sugar puts yeasts into total gluttony, leaving in their wake lots of nutrients.*

Once you have all these ingredients, the brewing can begin. The process can be broken down into three steps:

1. The yeasts break down the sugar.

2. The bacteria digest yeast byproducts.

3. The end results—kombucha brew.

The Yeasts Break Down the Sugar

Remember what yeasts need in order to survive? Organic matter. Carbohydrates. Sugar. That's right—the yeasts get their carbohydrates from the white sugar in the tea. You probably thought white sugar was bad for you. Generally you're right. Because it's such a simple sugar and can so easily be overused and quickly overload your body, white sugar probably isn't the best thing for our diets. But it *is* great for kombucha yeasts. After all, the yeasts need simple carbohydrates. And that's exactly what pure white sugar is. White sugar contains sucrose, a fairly simple carbohydrate—and no other "adulterating" ingredients that might be found in brown sugar, raw sugar, honey or other sweeteners.

So what do the yeasts do with all this "sinful" stuff? They eat it. The technical name for this process is "glycolysis," breaking down sugar.

Sucrose, the sugar in the tea, is actually made up of two even simpler sugars: glucose and fructose. Glucose is what the yeasts are really looking for. They gobble it up as quickly as possible. Other substances (enzymes) in the yeasts help process the fructose to make it more digestible to the yeast. As the yeasts break down the sugars, they leave behind plenty of ethanol (a type of alcohol), B vitamins, carbon dioxide and various acids. And as long as they're well-fed by any remaining sugar in the brew, the yeasts reproduce like crazy, enabling the entire brewing cycle to continue on and on.

Carbon dioxide given off by the yeasts mixes with the water and forms carbonic acid. These are the substances that give the "pop" to soda and the fizz to the kombucha tea. The ethanol—well, don't worry. It doesn't stay around long enough to give you much of a buzz.

The kombucha culture typically contains four main kinds of yeast: *Pichia fermentans*, *Kloekera apiculata*, *Saccharomycodes ludwigii*, and *Schizosaccharomyces pombe*. All four yeasts break down glucose. Each breaks down various other sugars as well. In addition to the kombucha culture, these yeasts are found in a variety of places ranging from buttermilk, olives and fruit to soil, flowers and oak trees.

The Bacteria Eat and Drink

The bacteria love the sugar, B vitamins and the ethanol. They suck up any sugar (glucose and the "treated" fructose) the yeasts don't manage to devour. Through the digestive process, they create the cellulose that makes up the kombucha culture's tough, slimy covering. And they slurp up the ethanol, too, creating acids as byproducts.

There have been more than 2000 types of bacteria identified in the world. Three of these are the main bacteria that live in the kombucha culture. Each has a different role in the brewing process, although their differing functions aren't well understood. In fact, it's only recently that the names of these bacteria have been standardized. Several older sources claim that many more bacteria were in the kombucha culture. As it turns out, a couple of different names were used to describe the same bacteria. Here's the list as it's currently understood:

> *Each type of bacteria has its own preferences for alcohol and sugar.*

- *Acetobacter aceti subspecies xylinum (Brown) comb. nov.* is the bacteria that is responsible for creating the cellulose "pancake." In addition, it eats the ethanol and oxygen and leaves behind acetic acid.

- *Gluconobacter oxydans subspecies suuboxydans (Kluyver and de Leeuw) comb. nov.* changes ethanol into acetic acid. It also creates gluconic acid.

- *Acetobacter aceti* gets most of its energy from the sugars left by the yeasts. It can also digest ethanol if there's also acetic acid available.

Acetic acid, the primary byproduct of the first two bacteria, is the same acid you'll find in vinegar. Other acids commonly identified in the brew and associated with the action of the bacteria include lactic, gluconic, oxalic and ascorbic (vitamin C) acids.

As the bacteria continue their binge and the sugar is used up, the yeasts slow down. Some of the remaining yeast buds latch on to the cellulose for safekeeping, until they find their next sugar fix—that is, when you start a new batch of brew. Others fall to the bottom of the brew, exhausted and dying.

What You're Left With

So once this process is complete, what do you have left? Here's a list, along with brief descriptions of each component.

ALCOHOL

A small amount of ethanol (usually about .5 percent) remains from the fermentation. The level of alcohol peaks about a week into the brewing

The fizz in the kombucha brew is caused by carbonic acid and carbon dioxide.

period and then starts decreasing after the end of the second week. And, yes, it's the same kind of alcohol you will find in a bottle of beer or glass of wine.

The alcohol content in the kombucha beverage, however, is typically .5 percent. Compare this with the 2.5 to 2.7 percent alcohol content of "lite" beer or the 3.3 to 9 percent alcohol content of the regular, full-alcohol versions of beer. The typical American lager is about 3.3 percent, porter can range from 6 to 7 percent and malt liquor tops off at about 5 to 9 percent alcohol content. When you compare these numbers, you can see right away that it would be pretty difficult to get drunk from the kombucha beverage. You could definitely call this stuff "kombucha lite" when it comes to alcohol content.

CARBON DIOXIDE AND CARBONIC ACID

As the carbon dioxide created by fermentation reacts with the water, it changes to carbonic acid. This is what gives the kombucha brew its carbonation. Carbon dioxide may also inhibit the growth of some contaminants.

GLUCOSE AND OTHER SIMPLE SUGARS

Depending on how much sugar you put in the tea, the yeast and bacteria may not be able to use it all up. Generally about 5 percent of the sugar remains unused and includes glucose, fructose and sucrose. Most of the sugar will probably be glucose. All three are simple sugars that your body can easily digest. But beware if you have diabetes or hypoglycemia: An unanticipated large hit of simple sugar can throw off your blood glucose levels. That's why many folks warn diabetics against drinking the kombucha tea.

If you feel you must try kombucha anyway (some anecdotal reports state that it has helped regulate blood sugar levels in some individuals), then make sure you let the brew ferment long enough to use up most of the sugar. Carefully monitor your blood sugar levels and adjust your diet accordingly.

B Vitamins

The yeasts and bacteria, as well as the tea itself, provide a range of the B vitamins, including B_1, B_2, B_3, B_5, B_6, B_{12}, B_{15}, biotin, folic acid, lecithin and PABA.

Vitamin C

Ascorbic acid is left by the bacteria's action and is also found in the tea itself.

Acetic Acid

Most of the alcohol in the kombucha brew becomes acetic acid, the same weak acid as is found in vinegar. The kombucha beverage may contain up to 3 percent of acetic acid. Because this acid is known to aid the growth of helpful bacteria and deter the growth of harmful bacteria (such as the food-poisoning substance *salmonella*), it's often considered to have a "detoxifying" effect on the body. But if the finished brew is left unused too long, acetic acid can react with any remaining alcohol to form acetates, which are strong solvents probably best left uneaten.

If the brew has an acetone-like smell—a sort of sweet yet caustic odor—don't drink it. Acetic acid can also react with cellulose, which is how rayon and film manufacturing begins. You probably don't have to worry about this happening to your brew!

Lactic Acid

Generally there is less than 1 percent of lactic acid in the kombucha beverage. Lactic acid isn't unique to the kombucha culture. It's a byproduct found in the fermentation process of any living cell. Like acetic acid, lactic acid may also be helpful in encouraging the good and discouraging the bad bacteria in foods and in the intestinal tract. It is also used by the body for energy.

GLUCONIC ACID

Not to be confused with the liver-produced glucuronic acid, gluconic acid does add some preservative value to the kombucha beverage. There's about 2 percent in the brew.

ENZYMES

Enzymes are a special type of protein that help cells generate energy. They are considered to be "catalysts," that is, substances that help energy generation without being used up themselves. Because of their ability to enable a range of chemical reactions, enzymes are used for food production, scientific applications and industrial purposes, such as baking bread, making antibiotics and creating rayon. In the case of the kombucha brew, the enzymes are contained in the yeast. In fact, the word "enzyme" (from the Greek) means "in yeast" or "leavening." It was only in the early 1900s that enzymes could be removed from yeasts and used for other purposes.

The enzymes in the kombucha culture include lactase and invertase. Each type of enzyme breaks down more complex sugars into simpler sugars, allowing the yeasts to continue their sugar feeding frenzy. Vitamin C and the B vitamins help the enzymes get started on their action. No one is completely sure, however, exactly how enzymes are able to effectively initiate so many types of chemical reactions without being "used up" themselves. Yet another wondrous biological process at work in the world around us!

AMINO ACIDS

Amino acids are the "building blocks" of proteins. When strung together in certain combinations, they form different types of proteins. Alanine, aspartic acid, esoleucine, glutamic acid, leucine, lysine, phenylalanine, serine, threonine, tyrosine and valine are all amino acids that have been reportedly found in the kombucha brew. A few others have been noted in yeasts in general, and are sometimes assumed to be in the kombucha brew as well. These include methionine, cysteine and cystine (the last two are derived from methionine).

OTHER SUBSTANCES

In addition to this list of the main byproducts from the fermentation and oxidation processes, you'll find small amounts of other compounds in the tea once the brewing is complete. Other acids may include tartaric, malonic (malic), citric, oxalic, and succinic acids. Little groups of yeast and bacteria may have broken off the culture and may be floating around in the brew (you'd probably have to get out your microscope to see them, though). The floating yeasts likely still contain some minerals. With the naked eye you may see some brown strands of cellulose. There is also some caffeine present (much less than what you'd find in the equivalent amount of regular coffee), as well as tannic acid, nitrogen and oxygen that didn't get completely used up in the brewing process. There are also lots of other compounds with long, scientific-sounding names that contribute to the kombucha brew's lovely odor and flavor.

Other Possible Components of Kombucha

There are other substances that may or may not be in the tea, depending on which source you believe. It starts to get tricky here, because the analysis of nutrients in foods is difficult and somewhat imprecise. In some chemical testing procedures, you have to know what you're looking for in order to test for it and possibly find it. It's not always possible to simply hand a bottle of unknown liquid to a lab and ask them to figure out everything that's in it. In addition, it's likely that different kombucha cultures have different components. After all, kombucha is a living, growing, changing organism. And with kombucha, like any good trendsetter, much of what seems to be "true" only becomes so because of repetition from source to source, not necessarily because of detailed investigation.

In any case, I will describe two of the substances that have been reported—but not necessarily consistently documented—to be in the brew. The only documented scientific statement about these components is from a scientist who emigrated from the former Soviet Union and wishes to remain anonymous. Unfortunately, this makes it difficult to

verify his information. You can read his complete statement in Günther Frank's book (see Resources section at the end of the book). The
following two substances supposedly have the greatest effect on your
health and are often the most highly touted components of the kombucha beverage.

GLUCURONIC ACID

This liver-produced acid grabs toxins in your body and shuttles them
out through your urine. This acid is one of the components of heparin,
which helps keep blood "thinned" to the appropriate level. In fact,
heparin and similar medications are frequently used to help keep
blood clots from forming in the body. Glucuronic acid also plays a part
in the development of collagen fibers, which form the skin.

USNIC ACID

Found in some lichens, usnic acid has antibiotic properties. It may also
prevent tumors from growing.

Kombucha's Not from Outer Space

Is all of this still sounding like a strange science fiction movie? A series
of unknown substances oozing out from a beige culture, bringing
peace and happiness to the world . . . . It's really not so unusual when
you think about it. Kombucha isn't the only weird fungal-bacterial
being fermenting out there somewhere. There are examples of similar
foods using these same processes from all around the world. Kefir,
yogurt, soy sauce, kim chi and even sauerkraut all rely on a similar
vinegar-like fermentation process. If you stop and think for a moment
or two, you can come up with all kinds of foods and beverages you
consume regularly that rely on similar processes: Bleu, Camembert
and Roquefort cheeses, wine, beer, leavened bread—even pickles.

But besides giving a tangy twist to your taste buds, what else can the
kombucha brew do for you? It's time to take a look at the purported
claims of many kombucha brew aficionados.

4

WHAT ABOUT
THE HEALTH CLAIMS?

_____

"My friends think I'm nuts . . . but they're the ones with plastic fingernails glued over their real ones."

"The latest underground information warns that the 'mushroom' is a sophisticated plot mass-marketed to poison people interested in self-healing. Supposedly the tea affects the brain. There is a slow degeneration of one's thinking and rationalizing processes . . . . After a short period of euphoria and increase of energy, the effects subside into depression. Many people have committed suicide . . . . If you are interested in healing, pass the word that the mushroom tea is a fabricated plot to make us sick, dependent and dead."

—Comments from the America Online
Kombucha Message Board

"My parents have been drinking the tea for months. My dad has fewer problems with dry eyes."

—From a conversation with a friend

So are any of these claims about kombucha's amazing health benefits or risks true? Or are they just hoaxes? And even if kombucha has some general "tonic" effect, what causes it? Could it be all the nifty vitamins and other ingredients created by the kombucha culture? Or are the millions of kombucha drinkers feeling better simply because of a sugar buzz or a caffeine high from the black tea?

Too many people have noticed too many positive effects from drinking the kombucha beverage for it to be total quackery. But realize that there is very little current "scientific" research into its health claims. Although there have been active periods of writing about kombucha in scientific publications in the past, I've chosen not to rely on them for this book. If you can track down the old articles, they make for interesting reading, but it's hard to verify their accuracy.

That leaves us in a tenuous situation as far as claims about kombucha are concerned. But it's not merely a problem with kombucha itself. In fact, it's hard to conduct good research to establish effectiveness for many health therapies. Just take a look at one health claim: Vitamin C reduces your risk of cancer. The only way you can definitively prove such a theory is by conducting a "double blind" study. That means everything is the same between two groups of people in the study, except one group receives vitamin C, while the other group receives a "placebo," something that is not going to affect them one way or the other. Neither group has any clue about whether they're taking the vitamin C or the placebo. Nor do the researchers know. Ideally, such a study should take place over a long period of time with a large group of people who represent the general population. Those are a lot of factors to try to control.

Here's another problem that has occurred with vitamin C research: Many of the studies review health records, have participants fill out surveys, or compile results from other studies that have researched the vitamin's effectiveness with a small group of people on a limited scale (such as men over 50 who smoke). So far from these compilations, no one can really tell whether or not people actually benefitted from the vitamin itself. They may simply have had lower rates of cancer because people who tend to eat a lot of vitamin C also tend to eat more fruits and vegetable and less fatty meats, all of which have also been associated with a reduced risk of cancer. You can see this whole question about whether a substance has been proven to be effective or not just isn't an easy one to answer.

Nevertheless, most documented benefits of drugs, vitamins or other health treatments begin with simple observations, long before the scientists get the grants from the National Institutes of Health to do research such as an official double-blind study. These simple observations—or anecdotes—cannot by themselves prove that something's beneficial, but they sure can make you wonder. And they can indicate trends that need further investigation. So, what about those anecdotal claims for kombucha's effectiveness?

The Claims

Positive changes from drinking the kombucha brew are usually noticeable within a month or two, according to most kombucha beverage drinkers' experiences. Generally, the brew's acidic contents should make your body digest food better. But don't despair if this is kombucha's main benefit to you. Better digestion is worth a lot—and can lead to all sorts of related health improvements. Traditional and alternative health practitioners both agree that better digestion can make you feel better and more relaxed. It can even make you look younger—with fewer wrinkles and a more glowing appearance. Others take it one step further: The "Kombucha Queen" herself, Betsy Pryor (founder of Laurel Farms), claims that the kombucha beverage's effects are spiritual, not physical or medical.

In any case, here's a list of all the benefits that kombucha beverage drinkers have reported. This list has been compiled from published research, published testimonials and unpublished conversations I've had with people who are actually drinking—or know someone who is drinking—the beverage on a regular basis. I've listed them according to frequency of report with the most commonly reported claims starting the list.

INCREASE IN ENERGY

The most frequent report from kombucha beverage drinkers is a feeling of overall increased energy or "feeling young again." Related to this claim is a need for less sleep and a decrease in insomnia. Others notice an increase in their sex drive or even a reduction in jet lag when traveling.

"BETTER" SKIN

Many people claim a variety of benefits to their skin after drinking the kombucha beverage. These effects include skin that looks clearer, appears younger and has fewer wrinkles and less cellulite. Others assert that drinking the kombucha brew has actually cleared up problems such as psoriasis and acne. Still others note the disappearance of liver spots.

IMPROVED HAIR QUALITY

Another common benefit claimed by kombucha brew sippers is an improvement in the quality of their hair. This includes thicker hair, the disappearance of gray hair, quicker hair growth, a slowing of hair loss and even some growth of new hair in formerly thin or bald spots.

IMPROVED NAIL QUALITY

Kombucha tea drinkers frequently notice stronger fingernails and quicker nail growth soon after beginning to drink the brew.

WEIGHT LOSS

Two common—and related—claims about the benefits of kombucha beverage include weight loss and reduced fluid retention.

LESS PAIN

Those who have routine pain due to arthritis, muscular aches or migraines often find that the pain is relieved after drinking the kombucha beverage. Similar benefits, as well as a reduction in numbness, have been noticed by people who have multiple sclerosis (MS), a disease that causes the nervous system to degenerate gradually.

BETTER DIGESTION

Benefits experienced by many who have tried the kombucha brew include more regularity in bowel habits, generally improved digestion and less pain from hiatal hernias.

DETOXIFICATION

Many kombucha beverage drinkers report a general body "detoxification" (which can include some unpleasant side effects such as nausea).

BETTER BREATHING

People who have allergies, asthma or upper respiratory problems frequently report that after drinking the brew they breathe easier and notice a reduction of asthma and allergy symptoms.

IMPROVEMENT IN CARDIOVASCULAR PROBLEMS

Several kombucha brew drinkers report a range of benefits associated with an improvement in heart or artery problems. These include less trouble with blood clots, a reduction in blood pressure and fewer chest pains.

LESS RELIANCE ON HARMFUL SUBSTANCES

Folks who previously relied on harmful substances such as alcohol to get them through the day often notice that after drinking the kombucha brew, the desire for alcohol, drugs, caffeine and even chocolate lessen.

SPEEDS HEALING

Several users of kombucha have noticed that cuts, scrapes, burns and cold sores tend to heal faster than before they drank the beverage. Some people even apply the brew directly to the wounded area. Others place a kombucha culture itself on the damaged area.

IMPROVED MENTAL HEALTH

A reduction in feelings of depression and anxiety has been noted by several kombucha brew drinkers.

REGULATION OF BLOOD GLUCOSE

Some people suffering from diabetes or hypoglycemia claim that it has been easier to stabilize their blood glucose levels when they drink the tea regularly.

FEWER PROBLEMS WITH PMS AND MENOPAUSE

Some women report that after drinking the kombucha brew, they have had a decrease in symptoms such as hot flashes and depression that are commonly associated with menopause. Others claim a decrease in premenstrual symptoms such as headaches, bloating and irritability.

DECREASE IN EYE PROBLEMS

A few kombucha tea drinkers mention that problems with "dry eyes" have resolved since drinking the brew.

IMPROVED IMMUNE SYSTEM

Several folks who drink the kombucha beverage claim an increased resistance to HIV infection and cancer. Some people with full-blown AIDS report a boost in T-cell levels. There are accounts of people whose cancer disappeared after drinking the brew. Others report that the tea has helped lessen the side effects of their cancer treatments, especially chemotherapy.

After reviewing this rather lengthy list, you may be wondering, "Is there anything the kombucha brew can't do?" Remember that these are listed according to frequency of mention in testimonials and anecdotal accounts collected in the kombucha literature over the years. None of these claims have been formally documented. For most kombucha beverage drinkers, the benefits usually include more energy, changes in fingernail and hair growth and, possibly, weight loss.

The Side Effects

Side effects, if felt at all, usually develop only when you first start drinking the beverage. That's why you should always start with only one or two ounces in the morning, and then slowly increase the amount to four ounces (½ cup). Here are some side effects that have been noted by others.

CONSTIPATION

Constipation is probably the most frequently mentioned side effect. It usually occurs when a person first starts drinking the kombucha beverage. You can avoid this problem by making sure your diet is high in fiber and that you drink plenty of other fluids throughout the day. Some folks also suggest that if you brew the beverage a few extra days or use multiple cultures in the brew, constipation becomes less of a problem.

"DETOXIFYING" EFFECTS

It's not at all uncommon to feel some nausea, dizziness and diarrhea, and to experience a change in urine color when first starting to drink the tea. Many alternative health practitioners attribute these symptoms to kombucha's detoxifying effects—it's ridding the body of some accumulated crud, which never feels great. If you notice these symptoms for more than a day, cut back or stop drinking the beverage.

Other Effects

Although these reports are rare, some folks have noted kidney pain, shortness of breath, rashes, lethargy and cysts. If you notice anything uncomfortable or painful, stop using the kombucha brew.

RESISTANCE TO ANTIBIOTICS

Although no cases have been reported, some health care providers are concerned that drinking the kombucha brew for a long time may cause you to develop a resistance to antibiotics. This theory (and it is only a theory) equates drinking the tea with overusing antibiotic medications, a growing problem that could dangerously imperil humankind. The difficulty with this theory is that, so far, no one has shown that the kombucha brew contains antibiotics, per se. The antibiotic effect may be due to other factors, such as the ability of some substances in the kombucha brew to prevent the growth of certain kinds of dangerous bacteria. In any case, some people deal with this possible problem by drinking the kombucha brew for a few months, stopping for a few months, then starting again.

ALLERGIC REACTIONS

Some people who are allergic to penicillin report having a similar allergic reaction to the kombucha beverage. Also, if you have a yeast allergy, it's probably a good idea to avoid drinking the kombucha brew, even though I could find no reports of allergic yeast reactions.

DEVELOPING AIDS

There have been a few reports of people who are HIV positive developing full-blown AIDS after drinking the kombucha brew. As far as I can determine, these reports are undocumented. However, it seems likely that anyone with a weakened immune system could experience negative reactions if there are any contaminants in the kombucha beverage.

At this point, no one knows whether any side effects are due to the kombucha beverage itself—or due to contamination of the beverage. In any case, if you notice any kind of negative effect, stop drinking the brew or at least substantially reduce the amount you drink.

What's Reasonable to Expect from Kombucha?

Will drinking the kombucha brew do you any good? Nobody has a definitive answer for you. In general, the kombucha brew is so acidic that it should be difficult for contaminants to grow—as long as you start with a pure culture and use proper brewing techniques.

But what is it about kombucha that leads so many folks to claim such a range of health benefits? Could it all be psychological? After all, taking any step to improve yourself can pay off big in terms of your sense of well-being. And there's nothing wrong with that. But maybe there's more to it. For instance, many kombucha beverage drinkers are older and seem to benefit greatly from drinking the brew. This makes some sense. The kombucha beverage contains many vitamins, minerals and acids—nutrients that everyone needs. The older you get, the more difficult it is for your body to absorb all these substances. That means you probably need even more in your diet. Drinking the kombucha beverage may simply be filling a nutritional deficiency. On the other hand, some kombucha advocates warn against trying to analyze the components of kombucha too closely. Rosina Fasching discourages looking at each individual component of the brew. She warns, "the whole is greater than the sum of its parts."

Fasching may be right. But it's still fascinating to see how some of the components of kombucha may contribute to the positive claims made about the brew. Let's take a closer look at some of the components identified earlier. This time, I'll focus on the health benefits associated with each. Please note that some of these benefits are *associated* with the substance, but may not be caused by the substance itself. For example, there's one school of thought that believes the benefits attributed to vitamin C and the B vitamins may really come from eating lots of fresh fruits and vegetables and less fatty meat. But even with that caveat in mind, it's clear that the substances found in the kombucha beverage may have a lot to offer.

Yeasts

Yeasts generate the brewing process, which results in nutritious byproducts. They also contain substances (histamine and tyramine) within their structure that can lower the blood pressure and the heart rate, although the amounts needed to do this are much higher than what you'd find in a typical dose of the kombucha brew. Yeasts may help with digestion, but too much yeast can lead to more harm (potentially to the liver and kidneys) than good. However, there is some evidence that a type of yeast found in beer—similar to the yeasts found in the kombucha brew—may prevent cancer cells from spreading to other parts of the body. And factors derived from yeasts have been used to speed wound healing. Yeasts also provide many of the amino acids and vitamins described below.

Acetic Acid, Lactic Acid and Other Acids

These acids have a range of potential benefits, many of which have been established by investigating the kombucha brew's cousin, vinegar.

These acids are often considered to have a "detoxifying" effect on the body. Acetic and lactic acids deter the growth of harmful bacteria—as evidenced by their use as food preservatives. Acetic acid has been shown to deter the growth of *salmonella*, the most common bacteria responsible for food poisoning. Acetic and lactic acids, as well as some of the other acids, also seem to have the ability to prevent certain other dangerous bacteria from growing in the brew. For example, one investigation showed that the kombucha brew was effective against *Staphylococcus aureus*, a common pathogenic bacteria that is responsible for staph infections, food poisoning and other ills. In fact, within the food industry there's a growing interest in using these kinds of acids to preserve foods, rather than relying solely on compounds such as nitrites that may retard spoilage but may give you cancer or other health problems.

In addition to inhibiting dangerous bacterial growth, these acids have other benefits. They can inhibit the growth of dangerous molds. They may encourage growth of "friendly" bacteria in the intestinal tract. Lactic acid gets shuttled from one part of the body to another in order to provide continuous energy for your muscles. It also gets converted into glucose, a simpler and easier energy source for the body to use.

Citric acid, like vitamin C, helps prevent scurvy. Malic acid may help prevent muscle aches. Oxalic acid helps your cells generate energy (but too much of it may cause kidney stones and gallstones to form).

All these acids may also have a slightly diuretic effect on the body, flushing out excess fluids and, hopefully, any toxins that are in the fluids. This not only provides a detoxifying effect, but may also cause some weight loss by reducing water retention.

> Your body puts together more than 20 amino acids in various combinations to build a range of proteins.

Amino Acids

One of the acids commonly found in yeasts is methionine. If methionine is, in fact, in the yeasts that reside in the kombucha brew, then we all have cause to celebrate. This acid and its two derivatives can help protect the body from pollutants and heavy metals such as aluminum and lead. Methionine is also known to help prevent cancer.

What else do you have to gain from the amino acids in the brew? Although more than 50 amino acids have been identified in the world around us—and all animal and plant proteins are made up of between 25 and 30 of these acids—you need to eat exactly eight of them on a regular basis to survive as a living, breathing human being. Why don't you need all 20-something? Your body can find a way to synthesize or create the others. The remaining eight are the ones your body can't derive from other sources, leading to their name, "essential amino acids." They include methionine, leucine, isoleucine, valine, lysine, threonine, tryptophan and phenylalanine. Most of these eight amino acids are in the kombucha culture. But the catch is you need all eight—within a reasonable time of each other—for the acids to form the proteins your body needs. This means that you can meet some—but not all—of your amino acid/protein needs from drinking the kombucha brew. In other words, don't go on a diet existing of only the kombucha beverage. You won't last long. Nothing substitutes for a well-balanced diet. The kombucha beverage is simply one more option to add to your food list.

Beyond forming proteins inside your body, amino acids have other purposes. Some amino acids are used directly to supply energy. Some help other substances found in the brew work more effectively. One good example of this is methionine, which enhances the activity of vitamin B_6. And, finally, you have some of these acids to thank for bringing you such a lovely smell as the kombucha brews. But besides providing the characteristic tart odor and taste, it's clear that the amino acids in the kombucha brew provide you with many potential benefits.

Vitamin C (Ascorbic Acid)

Like the eight essential amino acids, vitamin C is a substance that your body can't manufacture itself. But even though it's readily available in fruits and vegetables (one orange a day would do it), about half of all Americans don't get the daily minimum intake of vitamin C. Many of us should probably be getting even more. Smokers deplete their vitamin C supplies rapidly. And it appears that men, as they get older, need to increase the amount of vitamin C they eat. All this adds up to some basic advice: Don't forget to eat your fruits and veggies. And maybe the vitamin C in the kombucha brew can help you meet your vitamin C quota.

But why all the fuss about vitamin C? It won't prevent you from getting a cold, but it will help you get over it faster. Vitamin C has also been shown to lessen related symptoms, such as those caused by allergies and respiratory tract infections, including acute bronchitis and pneumonia.

Vitamin C prevents scurvy, a disease that once commonly caused sailors to die while out at sea because their diet lacked fresh fruits and vegetables. The symptoms of scurvy include bleeding gums, bleeding under the skin, slow healing of wounds, general weakness, loss of teeth, fatigue and depression. Sounds serious, doesn't it? In fact, the person who discovered how to synthesize vitamin C (Nobel Prize–winner Albert Szent-Gyorgyi) claims that many people have "hidden scurvy"—a vitamin C deficiency that causes no obvious symptoms, but which can lead to other health problems. This deficiency is easily cured by taking more of the vitamin.

Other reasons to maintain an adequate intake of vitamin C include the fact that the vitamin aids in the manufacture of collagen, a protein that helps provide structure to your bones, muscles, blood vessels, skin and cartilage. Vitamin C also keeps your teeth strong, helps prevent and cure periodontal (gum) disease and helps your body absorb iron.

There is substantial evidence that vitamin C boosts your immune system and helps lower your risk of cancer, especially in the throat, mouth, pancreas and stomach, and possibly in the cervix, rectum, lungs and breasts. Vitamin C may also relieve cancer symptoms, allowing people with terminal cancer to experience a higher quality—and longer—life. It has been used to help alleviate symptoms of some types of potent cancer-fighting drugs, such as adriamycin and interleukin-2. Some people think vitamin C should even be used as an anti-cancer drug itself, although the evidence is still unclear. And vitamin C may also protect against cancer-causing food additives such as nitrates and nitrites, which are found in processed meats such as bacon, bologna, ham and sausage.

New studies are pointing out vitamin C's ability to lower blood pressure (especially in people who smoke) and prevent artery disease. The way vitamin C lowers blood pressure is still unknown. Vitamin C's ability to prevent artery disease may be due to its strengthening the blood vessel walls and preventing too much low-density lipoprotein (a substance commonly called "bad" cholesterol) from clinging to the walls. Higher levels of vitamin C are also associated with higher levels of high-density lipoprotein (the "good" cholesterol) and lower levels of triglycerides (a fat found in blood also linked to artery disease), although the exact relationships are still not understood. And vitamin C may also cause the blood to be less "sticky," lessening the chance of heart attacks and strokes.

If you smoke, vitamin C can be depleted quickly. You need plenty of it just to maintain a baseline level of health but also to help counteract the damage cigarette smoke does to your body.

It seems that vitamin C can also affect sperm. Apparently the fluid that sperm swim in contains high amounts of this vitamin. Increasing an infertile man's intake of vitamin C improves his sperm's quality and motility (the ability to move around). This is especially true if the sperm clump together, rather than swimming individually. Improvements were even greater for infertile men who smoked. And the benefits may go beyond simply getting sperm to swim straight toward an egg. Undamaged sperm may mean fewer genetic problems—such as leukemia and certain other types of cancers—for the children created from the sperm.

Other research shows that vitamin C can block ultraviolet (UV) rays when applied to the skin—and it may also reduce the effects of aging on the skin. In one study, the effects lasted three days and the preparation didn't wash or sweat off, like normal sunscreens. Plus, vitamin C still allowed the sun to react with the body enough to generate vitamin D, something sunscreens currently on the market can't do.

What else can vitamin C do? There's more. How about prevent cataracts. If you were to measure it, you'd find lots of vitamin C in your eyes. It seems to protect both the lenses and the fluid that fills your eyes from too much oxygen and light. There is also some indication that vitamin C helps control (but not cure) glaucoma, a disease in which the pressure inside the eye rises dangerously high. It may also help prevent macular degeneration, another eye condition, in which an area of the retina at the back of the eye loses its ability to focus light properly.

How can vitamin C be so all-around beneficial? One reason is that it's an "antioxidant," a sort of natural preservative. You've probably heard about vitamin E and betacarotene as antioxidants—they've gotten most of the press up until recently. But vitamin C fits into this category as well—and, in fact, may be the most potent antioxidant of them all. That's why you'll see vitamin C or ascorbic acid in the list of ingredients of so many foods and drinks. As a preservative, it's cheap, it's effective and it's even good for you. However, antioxidants do more for you than simply preserve the foods you eat. Inside your body, antioxidants cause dangerous substances called "free radicals" to break apart or become inactivated before they can cause you any great harm. These free radicals are created in your body as a byproduct of burning energy. You're also exposed to them from outside sources, especially from air pollutants such as nitrogen dioxide, ozone, radiation and cigarette smoke.

About half of all Americans don't get the daily minimum intake of vitamin C.

Free radicals include individual atoms or small molecules of oxygen, iron and copper, among many other substances. They differ from regular, non-radical substances in that they have the wrong amount of "ions," that is, their electrical charge is different than what the substance normally prefers. That's why free radicals are so unstable. They're simply looking for a way to get back to their "normal" charge. But they aren't all bad. Your body needs a few of these unstable free radicals, some of which are used to help disable invading microorganisms. However, too many free radicals roaming through your body can create real trouble.

So how do antioxidants help control excess free radicals and minimize their damage? Let's take a look at how the antioxidant vitamin C deals with free radicals in your blood, thereby preventing artery disease (atherosclerosis), still the leading cause of death in the United States.

Your arteries are under a lot of stress. After all, blood is continuously flowing through them, pumped along by your heart. Once in a while the arteries become damaged—by accident, through bad habits like smoking or simply because of bad genes. When your body notices damage to the blood vessel walls, it calls in the low-density lipoproteins (LDLs), waxy substances that bring along the cholesterol that's needed to patch up the damage. That doesn't sound so bad, does it? However, sometimes the LDLs get a little carried away, rushing to the damage site in too great of numbers. As a result, they pile up along the blood vessel wall—without enough "good" cholesterols (HDLs or high-density lipoproteins) to drag them away.

Meanwhile, excess free radicals, unstable as they are, are also traveling around your bloodstream. They're in search of a charge—that is, an electric charge. They spy the piled up LDLs and decide they're the perfect solution! These radicals grab charged particles from the LDLs. The result? Without all their ions in place, the LDLs themselves become unstable. They actually "rust," a process called "oxidation," which is much like exposing bare metal to rain.

However, if you have substantial amounts of vitamin C in your body, you're in luck. Some is used for general body purposes, such as helping cells create energy. But the extra C floats around in your bloodstream, just waiting for something useful to do. That's why antioxidants like vitamin C are sometimes called "scavengers." These scavengers can search out and grab on to the excess free radicals and LDLs before oxidation—and major damage—can begin. They disable the free radicals and LDLs and carry them away to be processed and disposed of through your liver.

Some researchers have become so excited by this new understanding of vitamin C's role in heart disease prevention, that they now believe having adequate levels of vitamin C is as important as having a low cholesterol level or eating low-fat foods. Of course, no one knows yet just what an "adequate level" of vitamin C is, but it's an active research topic these days.

Oxidation caused by free radicals may also be responsible for other health problems, such as the spread of cancer and HIV (the virus that causes AIDS), damaged sperm, the development of cataracts and plain old wrinkled skin. And there's evidence that vitamin C, acting as an antioxidant, may be helpful in all these areas. But even beyond the role of vitamin C as an antioxidant, research continues into vitamin C's effectiveness in resolving other health conditions. Vitamin C may help the body use chromium to break down sugars, fats and proteins more effectively, especially in the elderly. The vitamin has shown some possibilities in reducing the pain and swelling associated with rheumatoid arthritis. It may slow down the production of a substance called sorbitol that is one cause of the complications associated with diabetes. Initial results in all these areas look promising.

Considering all these possible benefits from vitamin C, the claims made by Nobel Prize–winner Dr. Linus Pauling don't seem as far-fetched as they did when he first announced his belief in the power of vitamin C in 1976. His theory that vitamin C could add between 12 to 18 years to a person's life seems valid in view of the fact that Pauling himself lived an active and full life well into his mid-90s, continuing his research until his death in 1995. Besides, newer research—not just that conducted by the Linus Pauling Institute—backs some of the life-extending claims made for vitamin C. In any case, this is a potent vitamin that has so many positive benefits that it should come as no surprise that current research is showing that getting enough vitamin C can help you live longer. And, luckily for us, a source of vitamin C is the kombucha brew.

B Vitamins

It's likely that the kombucha brew contains most, if not all, of the B vitamins, since these vitamins reside in yeast. In general, the B vitamins help break down carbohydrates, proteins and fats into sugars so that your body can use the sugar for energy. Because of this central role, the B vitamins affect everything from your moods to the health of your heart. But the sad truth is many Americans are deficient in several of these crucial B vitamins. One study estimated 20 percent of older Americans have a vitamin B deficiency. In addition, it appears that you may need to increase the amount of some B vitamins you eat (such as B_{12} and folic acid) as you get older. Many health experts are so concerned about vitamin B deficiencies that they are reluctantly beginning to recommend multivitamin supplements. This is a big change for the nutrition and medical communities to make. In the past, they've been steadfast in the belief that it's best to get all your vitamin needs met through your diet, *not* through supplements.

The documentation of widespread vitamin B deficiencies may give us a clue as to why so many older people have reported substantial health benefits from drinking the kombucha beverage. It's possible that the brew is helping to make up for a vitamin B deficiency.

The substantiated claims about the B vitamins are many. Several of the B vitamins have been linked to relieving symptoms of depression.

Vitamins B_6, B_{12} and folic acid all play a role in maintaining clear arteries, helping to prevent heart attacks and strokes. They probably do this by regulating the level of homocysteine, an amino acid that is associate with increased levels of artery disease. When you're under a great amount of physical stress, you may need to increase the amount of B vitamins in your diet just to stay on an even keel. And B vitamins may be associated with glare-free vision.

The B vitamins have other individual benefits, as well. Here's the rundown.

Vitamin B_1 (thiamin) not only helps break down carbohydrates but also assists in maintaining your body's network of nerves. There is also some evidence that it, along with Vitamins B_2 and B_6, may reduce depression and related symptoms such as memory loss in older people.

Vitamin B_2 (riboflavin) aids in the breakdown of fats. It also helps cells use oxygen. And it's what might make your urine look more yellow if you start drinking the kombucha brew. Vitamin B_2 may also help lessen signs of depression in older people (see Vitamin B_1). And it works with vitamin A to prevent cataracts and eye fatigue.

Vitamin B_3 (niacin) has a range of benefits. It opens up your blood vessels. This might be one of the reasons it has been linked to relieving symptoms of arthritis: increased blood flow to affected joints may speed healing. Your cholesterol levels are regulated in part by B_3. Niacin and nicotinic acid—both names for vitamin B_3—are often prescribed for people with high cholesterol levels. B_3 is also involved in maintaining the health of your nervous system and in creating hormones.

Vitamin B_5 (pantothenic acid) may be the vitamin responsible for the claims that drinking the kombucha tea reduces gray hair. But more than that, B_5 is involved in almost every process your body undertakes.

Vitamin B_6 (pyridoxine) helps you digest and use proteins and fats. It also regulates the amount of sodium and potassium in the body in order to maintain correct fluid levels. Related to this benefit, is B_6's association with lower risk of artery disease. Along with vitamins B_1

and B$_2$, vitamin B$_6$ may also relieve symptoms of depression (see vitamin B$_1$). Vitamin B$_6$ is crucial for maintaining a strong immune system, your body's defense against invading organisms. Vitamin B$_6$ helps you develop the white blood cells you need to fight off infections. This vitamin may also play a role in maintaining healthy skin. Some physicians prescribe high doses of B$_6$ to relieve symptoms of carpal tunnel syndrome, which can cause tingling in the wrists and arms. However, too much B$_6$ can cause these very same symptoms. With all the potential benefits from an adequate intake of vitamin B$_6$, it's unfortunate that most people only get about half of the daily requirement of this critical vitamin.

> *It's likely that the kombucha brew contains most, if not all, of the B vitamins, since these vitamins reside in yeast.*

Vitamin B$_{12}$ helps keep the nervous system strong. For this reason, it's often recommended for people with Chronic Fatigue Syndrome (CFS, sometimes called the Epstein-Barr virus). Inadequate levels of B$_{12}$ are also linked with increased levels of artery disease, heart attacks and strokes. Not only can vitamin B$_{12}$ reduce the level of the artery-clogging amino acid homocysteine (homocysteine levels tend to rise as you get older), it actually changes homocysteine into methionine, an amino acid that helps prevent cancer. Vitamin B$_{12}$ (along with folic acid) has also been shown to reduce symptoms of depression, dementia, memory loss and confusion. It seems to enable people to think more clearly, even when they don't have a serious mental health disorder such as depression.

The problem with vitamin B$_{12}$ is, as you get older, it's more difficult for your body to absorb it, so you may need to increase your intake.

Vitamin B$_{15}$ (pangamic acid) helps your blood carry more oxygen.

Biotin, a B vitamin (but without a number), helps break down fats. It may also aid in the reduction of gray hair and hair loss. That's probably why you'll sometimes see biotin as an ingredient in hair shampoos and conditioners.

Many people would probably not need iron supplements if they consumed enough folic acid.

Folic acid (also called folate or folacin) is another numberless B vitamin that is now coming into its own. As recently as 1989, folic acid was not considered to be very useful, causing the National Academy of Sciences to cut the requirement in half. Even at this lower level, though, the average intake of folic acid is just over half the recommended level. But sentiments and recommendations about folic acid are changing as researchers discover more about its role.

You may already know that folic acid's primary function is to help your body use iron, which is essential for producing red blood cells. In fact, many people would probably not need iron supplements if they just consumed enough folic acid.

Folic acid has a range of other benefits, as well. Birth defects are reduced when expectant mothers have adequate folic acid intake. Women who are considering pregnancy are now being advised to take extra folic acid. (But remember, the kombucha beverage isn't recommended for pregnant women. They should find their folic acid from some other source, such as meat, fish, poultry, cheeses, grains, beans and leafy green vegetables.) Folic acid is crucial for maintaining the health of your arteries, and preventing heart attacks and strokes. Like vitamin B_{12}, it also converts artery-damaging homocysteine into cancer-preventing methionine. Some studies have shown folic acid to help prevent changes in the colon, cervix and lungs that could eventually lead to cancer. Getting enough of this vitamin can help reverse dementia, reduce symptoms of depression, enhance concentration, improve memory, and even simply help you think more clearly.

The amount of folic acid needed by your body may increase as you age. Even if you're younger, the role of folic acid is now considered to be so important that there is discussion about raising the daily amount of folic acid recommended by the United States Department of Agriculture (USDA). In the near future, the USDA may also require food manufacturers to add folic acid to breads, flours and other grain-based food products.

Lecithin (phosphatidylcholine or PC) is a fatlike, phosphorus-containing substance found in many plants and animals. If you look closely (with a microscope, of course), you'll find lecithin in your very own cells and in the coverings of your nerves. When you eat lecithin, your body breaks it down into several components: choline, phosphate, glycerol and some fatty acids. Once in the liver, these components are reformed into lecithin. Then the lecithin is distributed throughout the body, where it protects nerves and helps break down and get rid of fat.

There is also some initial evidence that lecithin may help alleviate symptoms of Alzheimer's disease. And due to its qualities as a polyunsaturated fat, theoretically lecithin should help lower cholesterol, although this benefit has never been proven.

PABA (para-amino benzoic acid) is more than just an additive to sunscreen lotions. Beyond absorbing the sun's ultraviolet (UV) rays, it helps your body produce folic acid and helps prevent gray hair.

Enzymes

Remember from our earlier discussion that the kombucha brew contains the enzymes invertase and lactase. Lactase breaks down lactose—milk sugar. Although there's not a lot of lactase in the brew, it still may be helpful to people who are "lactose intolerant," that is, folks whose bodies are unable to easily digest lactose. Invertase helps break down the sugar sucrose, which is why this enzyme is also called sucrase.

Glucose and Other Sugars

The simple sugars that remain in the brew can provide your body with quick, rich energy. However, as you've probably heard before, too much simple sugar simply isn't good for you. It can make your blood glucose levels rise and fall too abruptly, especially if you have diabetes.

Carbonic Acid and Carbon Dioxide

Your body produces plenty of each of these substances. However, if your body's processes are off a bit, the kombucha brew may provide just enough extra "oomph" to bring things back to normal. Once in the bloodstream, carbonic acid and carbon dioxide can join with sodium, potassium, calcium or magnesium to form "bicarbonates." These compounds are alkaline—the opposite of acidic—which is just what your blood likes. Order is restored!

Minerals

For such small creatures, the yeasts in the kombucha brew have a lot to offer. Minerals are just one more category of good things the yeasts bring to the kombucha brew. Again, don't forget that we're talking about yeasts in general here. We're making the assumption that this information transfers directly and accurately to the kombucha brew.

Chromium is a mineral that plays a role in regulating your blood glucose levels. Recent studies indicate that it may prevent artery disease and lower blood cholesterol levels. Chromium also helps build muscle tissue. Like several of the other nutrients we've talked about, many people are deficient in chromium. In fact, the USDA has determined that it's difficult for the average person eating less than 3500 calories a day—even when eating a well-balanced diet—to get the recommended amount of chromium. Since most of us eat less than 3500 calories a day, we're probably chromium deficient. So even if the kombucha brew contains just a little bit of this vital mineral, chromium is one mineral where every little bit helps.

Iron helps transport oxygen, carrying it through your blood and releasing it to all your body tissues. You'll find iron in many of your body's cells, including cells in your blood, muscles and other tissues. It forms a part of several enzymes that help your body generate energy.

Phosphorous works along with calcium to maintain your bones' growth and strength. It forms a part of many of the acids your body uses. It also assists in the breakdown of fats and carbohydrates.

Potassium is a mineral that helps regulate your body fluids, including your blood. Because of this role, it has a direct influence on your blood pressure.

Sodium is found in your body fluids. It is one of the things that keeps your fluid levels balanced. It also helps your muscles contract, powering your moves. Sodium is also partly responsible for making your nerves sense irritation.

Sulfur is needed in many parts of your body—in proteins used for hair, nails and cartilage, in the B vitamins thiamin and biotin, and in your liver for helping remove toxins.

Ergosterol

Ergosterol is a fatty oil, found most frequently in your skin. When sunshine hits this substance, it turns into vitamin D, which keeps bones and teeth strong by helping your body absorb calcium and phosphorus.

Caffeine

This substance suppresses appetite, leading to weight loss. That's why you find it in so many over-the-counter diet pills. But remember, the amount of caffeine in the kombucha brew is very low, so don't expect dramatic results.

Tannin (Tannic Acid)

This component of the tea medium may have some antibacterial effects of its own. At the very least, this acid helps keep bacteria or moldy contaminants from growing in your tea, a positive benefit to be sure. It also slows the fermentation process, which may account for the brew's low alcohol content. If you use green tea for brewing the kombucha beverage, you'll have a higher concentration of tannin than when using black tea.

Cellulose

There probably isn't a lot of cellulose floating around in the tea. But what is there is plain old fiber. And most of us are deficient in fiber in our diets. Fiber comes in two forms: soluble (dissolves in water) and insoluble (doesn't dissolve in water). Cellulose is insoluble—it's *not* the type of soluble fiber (such as oat bran) linked with preventing heart disease. Rather, insoluble fiber reduces constipation and speeds food through your digestive system more quickly. A related benefit is insoluble fiber's association with preventing certain types of cancer, especially cancer of the colon and rectum. The type of insoluble fiber most often studied and linked to cancer prevention is wheat bran. But since cellulose is one of the types of insoluble fiber found in wheat bran, it's likely that the cellulose in kombucha would have similar effects on your health. In fact, health practitioners generally recommend getting your fiber from a variety of foods, not just from loading up on wheat bran.

In addition to all the benefits described here, new health benefits for the nutrients found in the kombucha brew are being discovered and documented regularly. One example is a possible reduction of sudden infant death syndrome (SIDS) when infants receive adequate levels of vitamins C and biotin (a B vitamin). In any case, the list of benefits provided by the ingredients of the kombucha brew are impressive. And even if you decide not to try drinking the kombucha beverage, maybe this information will inspire you to search out other ways of getting enough of these nutrients on a daily basis.

What Does the FDA Have to Say?

Currently, there are no published scientific results about the kombucha culture and its brew from governmental agencies such as the United States Food and Drug Administration (FDA). The FDA has received many inquiries, however, and states that few problems have been recorded. One woman in Iowa did die after drinking the tea, but apparently she drank excessive quantities and had severe health problems. Most other reported problems have been linked to contamination. Researchers at the FDA are continuing to monitor kombucha use and will probably come out with more information in the future. In fact, they are currently brewing and analyzing the kombucha beverage and collecting information from state agencies about any reported problems.

According to Samuel Page, PhD, Director of the Division of Natural Products, the FDA's biggest concern is that people with weakened immune systems could have serious side effects from drinking a home-brewed kombucha beverage, especially if it contains any contaminants. The other concern, which led the FDA to issue a notice in June 1995, is that people brewing and storing the beverage should not use containers containing lead. This would include some ceramic and painted containers and lead crystal. The acids in the kombucha beverage can cause lead and other toxic compounds to leach out into the beverage. The FDA notes in the same bulletin that they have found no evidence of contamination in "commercial kombucha mushroom tea fermented under sterile conditions."

It's All a Matter of Perspective

"Vitamins are like seat belts. Wearing a seat belt doesn't give you a license to drive recklessly, it just protects you in case of an accident."

—Dr. Jeffrey Blumberg, Tufts University, in *Medical World News*

"Many people are bursting with good health and yet live at odds with themselves and the world. On the other hand, there are some who have been suffering from some illness for years . . . and yet they are the happiest people alive."

—Günther Frank, in *Kombucha: Healthy Beverage and Natural Remedy*

Blumberg and Frank hit the nail right on the head, and it's sensible to apply both their perspectives to all aspects of food and health, including the kombucha beverage. It looks like the kombucha brew contains many substances that can have great effects on your health. And many people report positive health benefits after drinking the beverage. But there's only so much one little fermented liquid can do. It's still up to you to develop and consistently maintain a healthy lifestyle—and to enjoy your life no matter what your health status. Maybe the kombucha beverage can become part of your ever-growing perspective on life, just like it has for millions of people for thousands of years throughout the world.

5

WHERE TO FIND KOMBUCHA

Kombucha use originated in Asia and then eventually spread throughout Russia and Europe. Today kombucha can be found in places much closer to home. If you decide you've simply got to try using this exotic culture, this chapter offers resources for locating already prepared kombucha teas and extracts, as well as kombucha cultures if you choose to brew your own.

Bottled Kombucha Beverage

It's interesting to note that the FDA has found no problems with commercially bottled kombucha beverages. That should help ease fears of many people who are worried about contamination. The bad news is that these bottled beverages usually are expensive. But if your time is limited and your budget isn't, bottled kombucha beverage may be a good solution. It's also a good way to try the beverage for the first time if you're thinking about locating a culture and brewing the tea yourself.

Bottled kombucha beverage can be found in many health food stores. Some stores have had problems locating suppliers of the beverage, so have taken to brewing it themselves. The demand for the beverage seems to vary widely from location to location—and you can't always find it where you'd expect it to be popular. For instance, I had a difficult time finding the beverage in Santa Cruz, California, usually a hotbed of health food trends and home to hundreds of alternative health care practitioners. Proprietors at a few health food stores hadn't even heard of kombucha but offered to put in a special order for me. On the other hand, my sister readily located the beverage in several small mom-and-pop health food stores on Florida's Gulf Coast. To avoid disappointment, try calling your health food store first to see if they carry the kombucha beverage.

Even though the FDA has found no evidence of contamination in commercially prepared kombucha beverages, before you grab a bottle of kombucha off the shelf, read the ingredients label carefully to know what you're getting. If it looks like a home-bottled venture, check with the health food store to see if they know anything about the bottler and the methods used. You could even take the extra step of checking out the bottler's facilities for yourself. In other words, beware of bottlers setting up shop in their garages or basements. They may have the best intentions, but preparing food for transport and sale requires strict adherence to sanitary practices, as well as meeting numerous federal, state and local requirements. You should also realize that some beverages containing the kombucha brew may have been treated with heat (pasteurized) to kill off contaminants. Heat probably also destroys some of the beneficial nutrients, especially the active yeasts and bacteria. But there's still probably enough good stuff floating in the commercially bottled brew to make it worth your while.

New sources of the kombucha beverage are popping up and old sources are disappearing all the time, so check in at your local health food store on a regular basis. Besides, if enough folks are asking for the brew, your store is sure to find a source somewhere. I've usually found the bottled beverage in the herbal preparations section of health food stores, not in the refrigerated beverage section.

There are two providers of the kombucha beverage that also sell their products through mail order. It's kind of curious that both distributors are located in Illinois. Who would have thought that the Chicago area would become the hub for kombucha distribution in the United States?

The largest supplier of the kombucha beverage is Pronatura. Their Kombucha Tea, imported from Germany, claims to use the "Genuine Dr. Sklenar®️ Recipe." The tea comes in 33.8 ounce bottles, which cost about $19.95/bottle.

Another provider of the kombucha beverage is Natural Choices. They began brewing the beverage for Sherwyn's health food store in Chicago—their operation is somewhat of a joint venture with Sherwyn's. Demand has been so overwhelming that Natural Choices started a mail-order business. They offer the kombucha beverage in one-gallon containers for $28/gallon. If you drink 4 ounces of the kombucha beverage each day, a gallon should last you a month.

Buying bottled kombucha tea, although expensive, may be a good way to introduce yourself to the culture. Just be sure to check out the source.

Another bottled beverage—the Yin Yang Harmony Drink, which has been pasteurized—also contains some kombucha extract, along with many other Chinese herbs. You'll usually find it with the refrigerated beverages in health food stores.

Kombucha Extract

Extracts are concentrated forms of a substance. The extracts you're probably most familiar with are those used to flavor baked goods: vanilla, almond and strawberry extracts, for example. Extracts are also made from herbs such as echinacea and goldenseal for medicinal uses. Kombucha can be made into an extract, too. The kombucha extract comes from the culture itself. Cultures are pressed, leaving behind a liquid filled with the culture's components: yeasts, bacteria and cellu-lose. Ethanol (grain alcohol) is added to preserve the liquid. The extract is then bottled. You use it by placing several drops in a glass of water, then drinking the water.

Kombucha extract can be a good alternative for people who simply can't tolerate the beverage's taste. It has also been recommended for people who have diabetes (the extract contains no added sugar) and for use when traveling or at work. The positive effects of the extract are generally similar to those gained from drinking the beverage, except more people report increased energy levels while taking the extract. In fact, many who use the extract claim that they can't take it too close to bedtime, or else it keeps them awake. But beware: You'll pay for the convenience of using the extract. Kombucha extract is much more expensive than the drink. You'll usually find the extract in the herbal preparations section of the health food store.

Pronatura offers the Original Kombucha Press Extract, Genuine Dr. Sklenar® Recipe. This extract is imported from Germany and sells for about $19.95 for a 1.69 ounce bottle or $29.95 for a 3.38 ounce bottle. If you follow the bottle's instructions and take 25 drops in water three times a day, the bottle will probably last you a few weeks.

Natural Choices also has a kombucha extract, made by Sherwyn's health food store in Chicago, which spent several months refining the recipe found in Günther Frank's book. The extract sells for $12/ounce, which should last about a week and a half if you take 12–15 drops two or three times each day.

Sources for the Kombucha Culture

If you decide you want to brew your own kombucha beverage, you'll need to locate a kombucha culture. Pick your source carefully: Make sure the culture was cultivated with the proper brewing technique and ingredients. You don't want to start off with a contaminated kom-bucha! That's one reason many people choose to pay the big bucks and order their culture by mail from a reputable vendor. But it's probably okay to get a culture from a friend as long as you check it out first. If you don't know anyone who is brewing the kombucha culture, ask at your local health food store to find local sources. Chances are that someone there will know someone else who is brewing the tea and probably has cultures to give away. Many health food stores even have bulletin boards for posting various health-oriented information. You're likely to find notices from people who are willing to give their cultures away. And we do mean *give* them away. Part of the kombucha tradition as it has developed in the United States is to never charge anyone for a kombucha culture. If someone other than a reputable mail-order company is trying to charge you anything more than postage, I'd keep looking. You may find the checklist below helpful when looking for a healthy kombucha.

The Healthy Kombucha Checklist

If your kombucha donor can answer "yes" to all these questions, you're probably going to end up with a healthy, uncontaminated kombucha culture.

- ❑ Does the donor know where the culture came from?

- ❑ Has the culture been brewed under clean conditions following techniques similar to those described in this book?

- ❑ Is the culture (not the "mother" culture, but the one your friend plans to give to you) less than a month old?

- ❑ Is the culture free of mold? (White wart-like bumps are okay, white or other colored cottony patches are not—that's mold.)

- ❑ Has the culture been kept safe from temperature extremes? Will it be kept safe from temperature extremes during transport to you?

Purchasing Kombucha by Mail

If you decide you'd rather purchase a kombucha culture from a commercial venture, here are two mail-order sources. These sources have been found to be reliable by many other kombucha brewers. For other commercial sources, talk to people you know who have purchased kombucha cultures from that source to find out if they're satisfied.

Günther Frank, the modern "father" of the kombucha tea trend, sells kombucha cultures for $50 (send a money order). Just remember that he's in Germany, so be prepared for delays.

> Günther Frank
> Genossenschafts Strasse 10
> D-75217 Birkenfeld
> Germany
> Phone: 011-49-7231-47810, Fax: 011-49-7231-485046

Laurel Farms is the largest U.S. distributor of kombucha cultures. Their cultures also cost $50. They sell the cultures at a reduced price to people with "catastrophic" illnesses such as cancer, multiple sclerosis and HIV/AIDS. Their phone line is a recorded presentation describing kombucha and giving you ordering information. If you order from Laurel Farms, you'll get a notice a few days before receiving the culture letting you know when to expect delivery and what to have on hand to start brewing the tea. The culture itself arrives U.S. Priority Mail, packaged in a cute little box with instructions that tell you, among other things, to "expect a miracle"—even though Laurel Farms makes it plain that in accordance with FDA guidelines, they can't make health claims regarding the benefits of the kombucha beverage.

> Laurel Farms
> P.O. Box 7405
> Studio City, CA 91614
> Phone: 310-289-4372

Natural Choices sells the kombucha beverage for $28/gallon. This price includes surface parcel post shipping, which usually takes 4–7 days. If you wish to receive the beverage more quickly, you can pay actual shipping charges (about $7/gallon). Natural Choices also has a kombucha extract for $12/ounce, shipped first class at no extra cost. If you call their phone line, you can order using Visa or Mastercard.

Otherwise, a check works just fine. Natural Choices doesn't take orders via e-mail but is happy to respond to any queries it receives electronically. I can vouch for their quick response time.

> Natural Choices
> 924 West Belmont, Suite #4
> Chicago, IL 60657
> Phone: 312-494-2695
> E-mail: nchoice@ais.net

Pronatura sells nutritional supplements and books on alternative medicine, including the books by Frank and Fasching. While most of their business is as a wholesaler to health food stores, they also fill retail mail orders. Pronatura carries kombucha products imported from Germany under the Dr. Sklenar® brand. These include the kombucha beverage ($19.95 for a 33.8 ounce bottle) and the kombucha extract ($19.95 for 1.69 ounces and $29.95 for 3.38 ounces).

> Pronatura
> 6211-A West Howard Street
> Niles, IL 60714
> Phone: 708-558-0900, Fax: 708-588-0918

6

HOW TO BREW AND BOTTLE KOMBUCHA

Brewing and bottling the kombucha beverage is the best choice for many people: it's inexpensive, it's relatively easy and—in most cases—relatively safe. Plus, it's kind of fun. However, it's scary to see how sloppy people can be in dealing with their kombucha culture. Like that childhood game called "gossip," as the baby cultures are passed from person to person, misinformation grows and valuable information gets lost. Many people simply hear about kombucha, inherit a culture from a friend (with no instructions), try to figure out what to do with the kombucha and then drink the brew they created. You could say it's a testimony to the antimicrobial effects of the acids in the kombucha beverage that more people haven't reported serious problems from drinking contaminated brew.

If you've decided that you're willing to do whatever it takes to brew kombucha yourself, welcome to the club. That's how most of us acquire our kombucha beverages. With a little bit of effort and the right materials, you, too, can be creating your own brew. It's not very hard and it should be safe—as long as you follow the instructions carefully. Read on for details.

Supplying Your Kombucha Brewery

You probably have most of what you need to brew kombucha right in your kitchen. In general, avoid supplies that contain metals other than stainless steel, such as aluminum. Otherwise, the metals can react with the acids in the tea and the culture. The most potentially dangerous metal is lead. If you use supplies that are glazed or painted, be sure the finish doesn't contain lead. Clear glass is generally your safest bet, although be sure it's not leaded crystal. If you're missing a supply or two—such as a glass brewing container or wooden spoons—DON'T SUBSTITUTE. Make the trek to your local store and get what you need. After all, you're planning to drink the stuff to maintain or improve your health. Why use the wrong materials and potentially contaminate your culture, your beverage, or you? Here's what you'll need to set up your brewery.

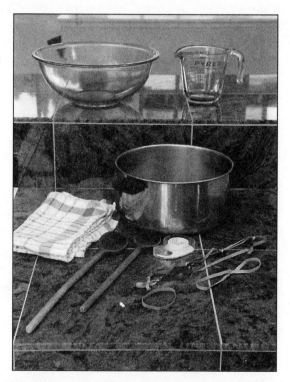

You probably have most of what you need to brew kombucha right in your kitchen. If you don't, make a run to the store. Don't make substitutions.

WHAT YOU NEED	WHY YOU NEED IT
4-quart glass, stainless steel or enameled pot	This container is used to boil the water and brew the tea.
Glass measuring cup, 1 cup or larger	You'll need this for measuring water and sugar.
Wooden spoons	You'll have to stir the tea occasionally as you add sugar.
Large 4-quart glass container	This is where the kombucha culture and tea will reside while they're brewing. Generally, it's advised to use a container with a fairly large opening so that the brew receives enough oxygen. A large glass bowl or a large, very wide-mouthed jar works. (If you're making a larger batch, you may even want to consider a glass aquarium.) Pyrex, manufactured by Corning, works well. If you can't find a good bowl at your local stores, call Corning Consumer Products directly at 800-999-3436, Monday–Friday, 8 a.m. to 8 p.m. Eastern Standard Time. They accept credit cards.

WHAT YOU NEED	WHY YOU NEED IT
1 cotton cloth	You need to cover the fermenting brew with something that allows air through, but keeps pests and particles out. An old T-shirt, flour-sack dish cloth (I buy these for about 50 cents each at the local drug store) or unbleached muslin (available for about $2.00 per yard at a fabric shop) will do. Whatever you use, make sure it's clean and free of holes. Cheesecloth is probably too loosely woven, allowing in small fruit flies.
Tape (optional)	I've found this tip from Laurel Farms to be helpful when using a very wide-mouthed bowl. Strips of tape applied across the top of the bowl keep the cloth from touching the brew.
Fastener for the cloth	You'll need to find something that you can use to securely fasten the cloth to the brewing container. This helps keep out flies and dust. I've found it easiest to tie together several rubber bands. You can also use twine or a large twist-tie.

WHAT YOU NEED	WHY YOU NEED IT
A warm, quiet, dark, well-ventilated place	The kombucha culture can thrive in temperatures ranging from 70 to 89 degrees Fahrenheit. The ideal range is about 70 to 77 degrees. Lower temperatures mean slower fermentation. Higher temperatures may damage the culture. So can sunlight. Ultraviolet (UV) rays can damage the yeasts and bacteria. A quiet place is helpful because disturbing the culture by moving it around too much slows the brewing process. I've found that an upper cabinet in my kitchen works well. It's out of the way, quiet, and warm enough for the kombucha to thrive. Plus the door keeps some of the vinegar-like kombucha brewing odors from wafting through the house, while still letting the kombucha receive enough air. Too little air will encourage mold growth. The last thing you want is that fuzzy stuff on your kombucha culture.

Ingredients

The ingredients for kombucha brewing are simple and, except for the kombucha culture and its starter liquid, readily available at any market.

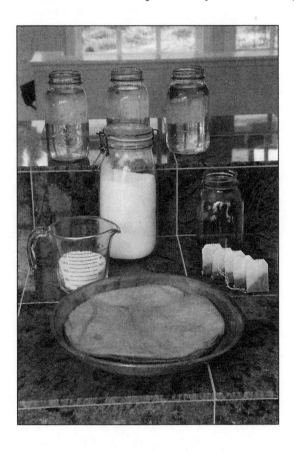

WHAT YOU NEED	WHY YOU NEED IT
2–5 tea bags	Black tea is preferable, since it has the best combination of nutrients needed by the kombucha culture. You can also try green or oolong tea bags in place of the black. Don't worry about the staples in the tea bags. They're small, the bags don't stay in the brew long and they never have direct contact with the acids in the fermenting culture. If you use loose tea, note that most tea bags hold about one teaspoon of tea. So, you'll need 2–5 teaspoons of loose tea. You may have to experiment a little to get the proportions right.
3 quarts of water	Distilled or filtered water is preferable. Water in most urban areas is treated with chlorine, which can damage the culture. Well water may be okay if it doesn't have added chemicals and if there aren't too many minerals in it.

What You Need	Why You Need It
1 cup (8 ounces) white sugar	Plain old white sugar is what you need. Honey contains substances that may inhibit growth of the beneficial bacteria in the kombucha culture. Other types of sugar (raw, brown, etc.) may contain impurities that could contaminate the culture. Sugar substitutes may be great for helping you lose weight, but they will cause your kombucha to starve to death.
1 kombucha culture	See the list earlier in this book for a source for the kombucha culture.
½ cup starter liquid or cider vinegar	Use the liquid that came with your kombucha culture (if this is your first batch) or unstrained liquid from your latest batch. If there's not enough or if you had to throw out a bad batch, use ½ cup of cider vinegar instead.

Ten Steps to Brewing Success

Brewing the kombucha beverage isn't hard. You just need to follow these ten steps. Don't be tempted to take shortcuts or rely on your memory alone. Every time you make a new batch, pull out these instructions to make sure you're doing everything correctly. Failure to follow the steps properly could lead to contaminating your kombucha culture or the brew itself. The consequences can be unpleasant and even dangerous if you drink the contaminated brew.

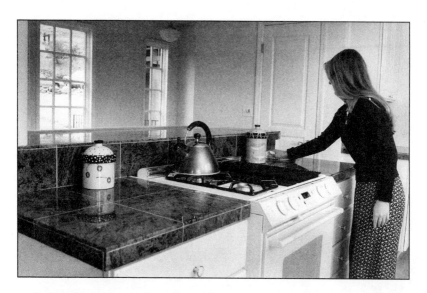

1. START WITH A CLEAN KITCHEN.

"Clean" means two things: spotless and uncluttered. You need to clean up any dirty dishes, counters and other areas of your kitchen that need it. You may be able to survive in a dirty kitchen, but the kombucha can't. Make sure you don't have potential contaminants lying around, such as fresh fruit or houseplants. These substances harbor less-than-beneficial yeasts and bacteria that would just love a chance to find their way into your kombucha culture. Clean also means that your hands have been washed and all equipment is spotless. If possible, wash everything in the dishwasher—just to be sure your supplies are as clean as possible. Hot dishwasher water should be able to kill off just about any microorganism lurking in the cracks or crevices of your supplies. Why all the fuss about cleanliness? It's not that I'm encouraging "godliness" per se, although that's a noble goal. It's just that most cases of people getting sick from drinking the kombucha beverage have occurred because contaminants somehow entered the culture or the brew. The brew is usually acidic enough to handle most of them. But if it becomes overwhelmed by an unwelcome yeast or bacteria invasion, you may suffer the results. Maintaining a clean brewing environment is an easy way to ensure that your kombucha brew stays uncontaminated—and that you remain unharmed.

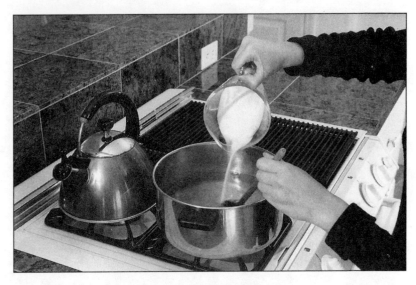

2. BRING THREE QUARTS OF WATER TO A BOIL. AS IT IS HEATING UP, STIR IN 1 CUP OF WHITE SUGAR.

Make sure the sugar dissolves into the water, and doesn't settle down at the bottom, where it can burn and release toxins of its own.

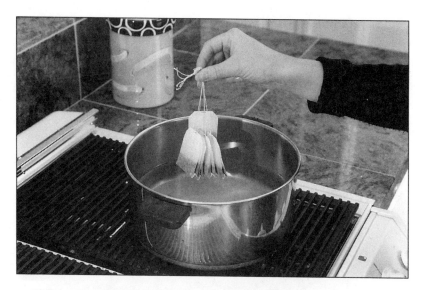

3. **JUST AFTER THE WATER COMES TO A BOIL, TURN OFF
THE STOVE AND REMOVE THE POT FROM THE BURNER.
ADD 2–5 TEA BAGS.**

Some sources recommend letting the water boil for 5 minutes. Others
say that boiling the water that long can damage the sugar. You'll have
to decide which technique works best for you. I pretty much split the
difference and remove the pot within a minute after the water comes
to a boil. That way I'm sure the water is sterilized, but the sugar hasn't
been unduly harmed. If you're using loose tea, put in 2–5 teaspoons.
Just drop it in the tea—without a tea ball or other infuser.

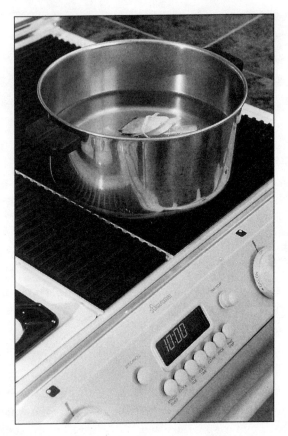

4. LET THE TEA STEEP FOR 10 MINUTES, THEN REMOVE THE TEA BAGS.

If you're using loose tea, you'll have to strain the tea after it has steeped for 10 minutes. In addition to the supplies listed above, you'll need a cheesecloth or a strainer. Metal is probably okay, since it will not be exposed to the culture or fermenting brew.

Slowly pour the tea through the strainer and into the fermentation container. After your first batch, you'll also need an extra glass container for your tea to rest in while it cools. You don't want to pour it right away into the bowl that has sediment in the bottom. This hot tea would kill the active yeast and bacteria in the sediment.

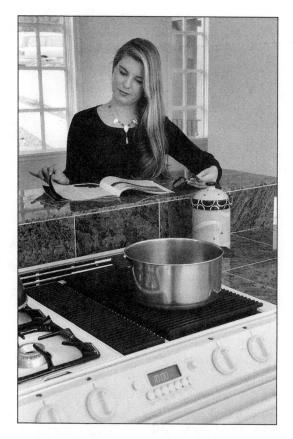

5. LET THE TEA COOL DOWN UNTIL IT IS BETWEEN LUKE-
   WARM AND ROOM TEMPERATURE.

It should take around a half-hour for the tea to cool to a lukewarm temperature. However much time it does take, don't move to the next step until the tea is lukewarm. Otherwise, the excess heat can damage— and even kill off—the yeasts and bacteria in the kombucha culture.

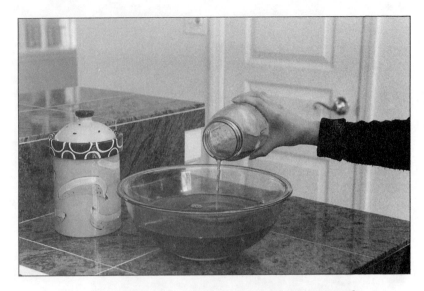

6. POUR THE TEA INTO THE FERMENTATION BOWL. ADD THE ½ CUP OF UNFILTERED "STARTER" LIQUID.

Don't forget the starter liquid! If you don't have enough, use cider vinegar. Otherwise, your culture will have a hard time revving up. Some sources recommend boiling the vinegar first. It seems, though, that this is overkill. The vinegar is so acidic that it's probably free of any contaminants. You'll have to use your own judgment on this one. If you're beyond your first brew, you can leave the yeasty sediment from the previous batch in the bottom of the fermentation bowl. Be sure to thoroughly clean the bowl, though, at least once a month. When I first started brewing the kombucha, I made the mistake of cleaning the sediment out of the bowl every time I brewed a new batch. As a result, my kombucha cultures were a little thin and wasted. Leaving the sediment seems to cause the brew to work more quickly and the cultures to grow more robustly.

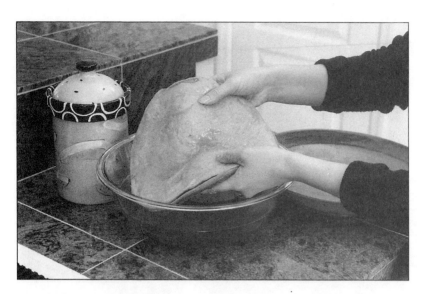

7. PLACE THE KOMBUCHA CULTURE ON TOP OF THE TEA.

The smooth, shiny layer should face up. The rough, darker brown layer should be down, resting on top of the tea. Don't be worried if the culture sinks to the bottom. It will probably rise up while the tea is brewing over the next week.

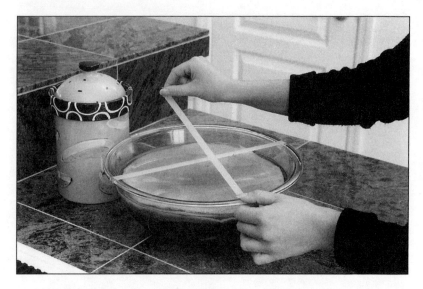

8. COVER THE TOP OF THE FERMENTATION CONTAINER WITH STRIPS OF TAPE.

This step is optional. If you use a container with a very wide mouth, the tape will help keep the cloth from sagging into the brew.

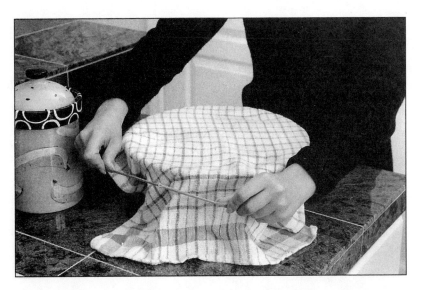

9. COVER THE FERMENTATION CONTAINER WITH A CLOTH. SECURE IT.

The cloth cover helps keep bugs, flies and other unwanted objects out of your tea. It still allows air in.

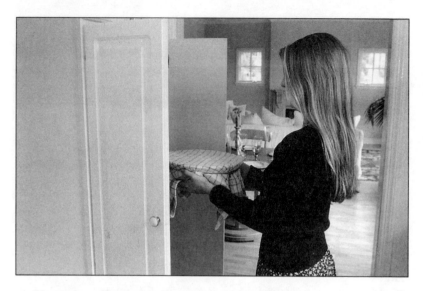

10. PLACE THE FERMENTATION CONTAINER IN YOUR "KOMBUCHA BREWING SPOT." LEAVE IT IN THIS SPOT FOR 5–10 DAYS.

Don't forget that the kombucha needs a warm, quiet, dim place so it can brew most effectively. Try not to disturb it for the entire brewing time. The ideal brewing period seems to be about 7–10 days. You'll have to experiment to find out how many days works for you. If it's warmer, you may need to leave the brew for only 4–5 days. If the weather's cooler, it may take more than a week. Generally, the shorter the brewing time, the sweeter the brew. I've found that even 8 or 9 days produces a brew that's too tart for my taste. In any case, after 10 days, there's probably not much sugar left to ferment and you'll have a very tart beverage chock full of nutrients.

Bottling the Results

It's quite exciting the first time you finish a batch of kombucha beverage and are ready to bottle it. But before you rush through the bottling process, be sure all your supplies are ready to go. And if you're planning to start another batch brewing right away (which I'm sure you'll want to do), get out the tea-making equipment before you get everything else underway. Again, make sure all your supplies are squeaky clean and your kitchen is free of potential contaminants.

Bottling Supplies

You'll need a few more supplies when it's time to "harvest" your kombucha brew. Most of these should be readily available in your kitchen. And don't make substitutions that could damage the brew or you. Even though the fermentation process will be substantially slowed, the liquid still contains lots of acids that could react with certain metals.

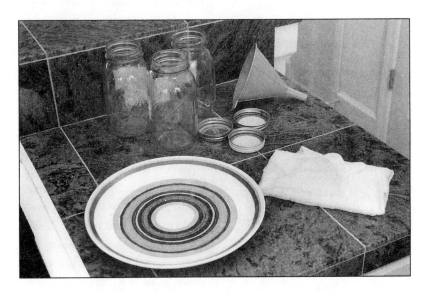

Bottling your first, foaming batch of brew is simple.

WHAT YOU NEED	WHY YOU NEED IT
Large plate	You need a plate that's large enough to hold your kombucha while you are straining the beverage and getting the next batch ready. Be sure to use a plate that doesn't contain lead in the glaze. Also avoid metals and leaded crystal.
Storage containers	Glass works best—most any type of glass bottle will do. The reason for using glass for storing the beverage is basically the same as for brewing the beverage. Even though you've removed the beverage from the active culture, you'll still find a few free-floating strands of yeast and bacteria. Some fermentation—even in the cooler refrigerator—is still occurring, although at a much slower rate. Most importantly, though, the resulting brew is full of acids that could cause lead or other metals found in glazed or metal containers to leach into the beverage—not a good additive to your healthful brew. I've found that one-quart canning jars work well for storing the brew. Just make sure the metal lids don't touch the beverage. If you want to get fancy, you can buy bottles and corks through a local beer- or wine-making supplier.

What You Need	What You Need
	Look under "Beer Home Brewing Equipment and Supplies" or "Wine Makers Equipment and Supplies" in your phone book's Yellow Pages. Or you can reuse empty glass jars from mayonnaise, sodas and other food products. Whatever you use, just be sure that you get both the jars and the caps exquisitely clean so there's nothing to contaminate your kombucha beverage.
Cheesecloth	This time the wider holes in cheesecloth will work. You use this cloth to strain the fermented kombucha brew.
Plastic funnel	You use the funnel to hold the cheesecloth while the kombucha beverage filters through.

Five Steps for Bottling Your Brew

You've been waiting patiently for about a week while your kombucha has been brewing. You've lined up all your bottling supplies. You're even ready to make a new batch of the brew right away. Now is the time you've been anticipating: Bottling the kombucha brew. Just follow these five steps and you're on your way.

1. **CAREFULLY REMOVE THE FERMENTATION CONTAINER FROM THE KOMBUCHA BREWING SPOT. TAKE OFF THE CLOTH AND TAPE. SAY "HELLO" TO A NEW KOMBUCHA CULTURE.**

It's likely that the kombucha is still floating on top of the container. You will notice that your old culture has an offspring. The new culture that formed during the brewing process sits on top of the old one. It may be totally separated from the original culture. In fact, the older culture may be resting at the bottom while the newer culture floats on the top. Or the newer "baby" may still be clinging to

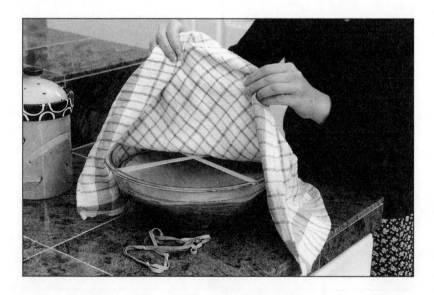

its "mother." To your surprise, you may find yourself getting somewhat sentimental over this wondrous event of nature. Watching the
babies grow is one of the things that makes kombucha brewing so
enjoyable.

2. REMOVE THE CULTURES FROM THE BREW AND PLACE THEM ON A CLEAN PLATE.

Remember not to use metal, leaded crystal or lead-glazed ceramic
plates—no heavy metals for you and your kombucha! If the kombucha
looks a little grungy, feel free to rinse it off in tepid water. The cultures
feel funny, don't they? Kind of hard and squishy all at the same time.
You'll probably notice that the younger culture is more fragile than the
older one. You can separate the cultures if you wish—give one of them
and the brewing instructions away to a friend. Or you can start two
batches at once. Or leave the cultures together for a bit longer (you'll
probably get still another culture with each batch you make). It's estimated that you can easily use the same culture for two or three
months—or even longer—before it runs out of steam.

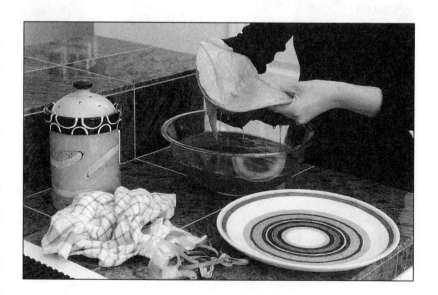

3. POUR THE BREW THROUGH THE CHEESECLOTH AND FUNNEL IT INTO YOUR CONTAINERS.

This is the part that, for me anyway, requires coordination. Straining the brew simply removes some of the clumps so that the beverage is easier to drink. The clumps are probably either dead or dying yeast clusters or mini-yeast/bacteria/cellulose packages waiting to become full-fledged cultures. While you're filling the bottles, you will notice that the brew now fizzes. This is due to the carbonic acid and carbon dioxide created during the fermentation process. It gives the beverage an extra refreshing zing. Fill the containers almost to the top. I leave just enough air space in the jars so that the brew doesn't touch the jar's lid.

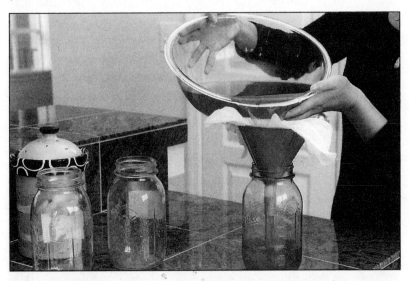

4. CAP THE BOTTLES AND STORE.

Some people leave the beverage out of the refrigerator in a cool, dark place. If you do this, realize that your kombucha brew will continue to ferment. Those clumps may even turn into full-fledged mini-cultures. Since the beverage is still actively fermenting, it will continue to change in taste, as well. It will become more acidic and vinegar-like the longer it sits. The other choice—and what most people do—is to put the beverage in the refrigerator. There, the fermentation process is seriously slowed by the cool temperature. You may still see some strands of culture, but not as much as if you left the brew out in the warmer environment. Because the fermentation process is slowed in the refrigerator, the beverage will pretty much maintain the flavor it has when bottled, maybe becoming just slightly more acidic if you leave it in the refrigerator for long.

5. Get started on the next batch of kombucha beverage.

Start your new batch by following the ten steps described previously.

Now's the time to take the first sip of your bottled kombucha brew. What do you think? Many people love it at first sip. Others aren't so sure. If you're in this second group, don't be too concerned. The taste of the beverage does kind of grow on you after awhile, sort of like drinking wine. As you get used to the brewing process, try experimenting with the length of fermentation until you find the amount of time that generates a brew you enjoy. Remember, though, that the time you need changes with warmer and colder temperatures. Brewing time will probably lengthen during the winter and shorten in the summer.

How much of this beverage should you drink? That depends. But start off slowly—probably with about 2 ounces (⅛ cup) per day. Gradually increase the amount you drink to 4 ounces (½ cup) per day. Most folks recommend drinking the tea in the morning before you eat breakfast. It seems to be a good way to get your body up and running quickly! Try it instead of that morning cup of coffee—and see if you notice a difference.

Most of us will probably limit our kombucha beverage intake to about ½ cup per day. Others may want to try more. If so, just be careful that you don't overdo it. After all, kombucha is supposed to be just one part of your overall healthy eating plan. You can't rely on kombucha alone for all the nutrients you need. You'll probably be okay drinking ½ cup before breakfast and then ½ cup with each of your remaining two meals. That's a total of 1½ cups (12 ounces) per day. Work up to that amount slowly. Otherwise, you may notice more unpleasant side effects. The goal is to help your body get healthier, not to make you miserable.

So what do you think? Brewing kombucha isn't so hard once you get the hang of it. And once it seems routine, you may want to figure out other things to do with the beverage—and with your ever-growing cultures. If so, we have some suggestions for you in Chapter 7.

7

HOW TO USE KOMBUCHA

Now that you've figured out how to brew the kombucha beverage, you have all these jars in your refrigerator. What are you supposed to do with them? Can you use up all the kombucha brew before your next batch is ready? You'll probably find that it disappears quicker than you'd expect. Many people have two or three batches brewing simultaneously, especially if their family or friends start drinking the kombucha beverage. Let's take a look at what you can do with all that liquid resting in your refrigerator. First, I'll give some information about how to drink the brew. Then I'll explain how you can use it in other fun ways—from cooking to personal hygiene to household cleaning.

Drink It

Practically everybody who has advocated drinking the kombucha beverage agrees that you should drink about 4 ounces (½ cup) of the kombucha beverage first thing in the morning. Most sources suggest you leave it at that. After all, you are dealing with a beverage that's chock full of vitamins and other nutrients. Like anything else, too much of a good thing isn't necessarily better.

So do yourself a favor and start with a small amount—maybe an ounce—to let your body get used to the tea. If everything seems okay, gradually increase the amount until you reach the 4 ounces. If you feel like you could benefit by drinking more of the kombucha beverage, increase the amount gradually, drinking an additional 4 ounces with lunch and with dinner.

On the other hand, what should you do if you just can't stand the way the stuff tastes? I don't really believe the advice I've seen in some of the on-line discussions that state you need it even more if you react badly to the flavor. Even if this were true, why force yourself to drink something you're only going to gag on? And if you haven't fallen in love with kombucha's flavor, you're not alone. Although some people immediately like the kombucha taste, others hate it. If you're not too impressed after your first few sips, keep trying to drink a small amount of it each morning, as long as you're not having side effects. Think of it like the first few times you tried to drink prune juice at your grandmother's house or the first time you attempted to act cool by sipping a beer without making a face. Gradually you begin to appreciate the flavors in these strange-tasting beverages and eventually you may even enjoy them!

However, even after many attempts you may find that your brew is just not your cup of tea. If so, consider experimenting a little with the brewing process—the number of days the brew ferments or the amount of sugar you use—to find the level of taste that works for you. The thing you have to realize, though, is you may be giving up some of kombucha's potential health benefits in order to please your palate. I, myself, have made this tradeoff. I'm not fond of overly tart kombucha, so I let it ferment only 5–7 days rather than the 8–10 days that many sources indicate is optimal for health benefits. If you decide you want to adjust the beverage, read on for suggestions.

If It's Too Sweet

- Try letting the culture ferment a few more days before you strain and bottle it. The longer the beverage ferments, the more sugar the culture uses up.

- If you're diabetic and worried about the sugar in the beverage, consider using the kombucha extract instead.

If It's Too Tart

- Try diluting it with water (distilled or filtered is preferable).

- Let the brew ferment one or two days less than the standard instructions. The shorter the fermentation time, the more sugar will remain in the beverage. Of course, that also means there will be fewer nutrients. But it's probably better to drink the kombucha beverage minus a few nutrients than to drink none of the brew at all.

- Add some freshly brewed black or green tea. But make sure the tea is pretty much at room temperature or cooler. Otherwise you may destroy some of the nutrients—the live yeasts and bacteria—in your kombucha brew.

- Mix in some apple juice or grape juice just before drinking your brew. Just remember: If you add anything to the brew, do it just before drinking it—and don't let it sit around for long. You don't want the culture to start interacting with whatever you poured into the beverage.

For a Change of Pace

- Add fresh fruit or preserves when drinking or bottling the beverage. Be sure not to let the fruit come into contact with the kombucha culture itself, or the culture may become contaminated. You know just how quickly fresh fruit can spoil. That's because it has lots of yeasts and bacteria hiding out on it. After you've strained and bottled the beverage, simply place a few pieces of fruit in the bottle. The brew takes on just a hint of the taste and color of whatever fruit you use. Try raspberries, blackberries, cherries, peaches, raisins or even fruit tree blossoms.

- Try adjusting your tea mix. Swap one or two black tea bags for some of the green tea. Or try a few bags of oolong tea, which is somewhere between green and black teas in terms of caffeine level and taste. It's probably a good idea to avoid herbal teas, unless you absolutely know that the oils in your favorite herbal blend won't react with the kombucha culture.

Cook With It

The kombucha beverage is great for drinking. But you can cook with it, as well. However, if you heat up the brew, you will lose some of the nutritional benefits, predominately from the yeasts. And if you use kombucha beverage in something that's not being cooked, be sure to keep the food refrigerated so the live yeasts and bacteria in the kombucha beverage don't start fermenting the food you've added it to. Keeping these two caveats in mind, go ahead and experiment! Use these ideas—and even some of the following recipes—to have your very own "kombucha tea party."

Kombucha as Condiment

Think of the variety of vinegars you can find in the grocery store: cider, wine, white, malt, flavored. Vinegars add a special taste to many dishes. The kombucha brew can serve much the same purpose. When the kombucha beverage ferments for a longer period of time, most of the sugar and alcohol are used up, increasing the amount of acid. The result is like a mild- to medium-tasting cider vinegar, with a somewhat sweet flavor that complements most foods well. Generally, you can use this as if it were vinegar, especially in marinades and salad dressings. But there's one exception: Don't try to preserve anything with kombucha vinegar. Unlike regular vinegar, the kombucha brew is still active and unsterilized. Who knows what your pickles would mutate into! If you want to try making kombucha vinegar, here's what to do:

1. Let an occasional batch of your kombucha beverage sit in its bowl for an few extra days until it gets really strong.

2. Strain, bottle and store the beverage in a glass container. You may also want to label it, too, or else you may get an especially tart surprise one morning when you grab the wrong bottle of your favorite wake-up brew.

KOMBUCHA BREW SLAW

¼ cup kombucha beverage

½ cup mayonnaise

¼ teaspoon each of dill weed, celery seed, black pepper and tarragon

Sugar to taste (optional)

½ head green cabbage

1 medium carrot

1. Stir kombucha beverage, mayonnaise, herbs and sugar together until well blended.

2. Shred cabbage and carrot and place in bowl.

3. Pour in kombucha dressing and mix well.

4. Refrigerate when not being served.

The dressing adds a nice sweet-sour taste to cole slaw that's not quite as strong as using regular vinegar.

KOMBUCHA PASTA SALAD

½ box or bag (6 ounces) of pasta, cooked according to the package's instructions

¼ cup finely chopped onion

¼ cup finely chopped celery

¼ cup diced sweet red pepper

¼ cup halved green olives

1 diced dill pickle

½ cup sliced zucchini

½ cup mayonnaise

¼ cup kombucha beverage

¼ teaspoon each of dill weed, tarragon, celery seed, oregano, pepper and salt

1. In a large bowl, mix the cooked pasta and vegetables.

2. In a small bowl, mix the mayonnaise, kombucha beverage and spices until well blended.

3. Pour the dressing into the large bowl and stir until the dressing is evenly distributed.

4. For optimal taste, chill for several hours before serving (overnight works well). Refrigerate when not being served.

For a variation, try adding shredded carrots, fresh or frozen peas, corn kernels, broccoli flowerettes or other vegetables—whatever you have on hand will probably work.

TANGY KOMBUCHA MARINADE

¼ *cup kombucha beverage*

2 *tablespoons soy sauce*

1 *teaspoon ginger*

½ *teaspoon garlic powder*

Pepper to taste

🐞

1. Combine all ingredients thoroughly.

2. Use to marinate vegetables, fish, chicken or beef
(the kombucha beverage quickly and effectively
tenderizes meat).

3. Grill, broil or bake, basting with the marinade
frequently.

KOMBUCHA BARBECUE MARINADE

¼ *cup kombucha beverage*

¼ *cup ketchup or tomato sauce*

1 *teaspoon Worcestershire sauce*

Pepper to taste

🐞

1. Combine all ingredients thoroughly.

2. Use to marinate shrimp, chicken, beef or ribs
(preferably overnight).

3. Follow your favorite grilling techniques.

4. When turning the meat, baste with more marinade.
Works well with *carne asada* (grilled, chopped steak)
or beef skirt steak.

SPICY GRILLED KOMBUCHA SHRIMP AND VEGGIES

½ pound large uncooked shrimp

1 zucchini

1 small eggplant

2 medium tomatoes

2 tablespoons kombucha beverage

4 tablespoons olive oil

3 teaspoons chili powder

½ teaspoon hot pepper sauce

2 cloves garlic, minced

½ teaspoon salt

1. Cut off shrimp legs. Remove vein by slitting along shrimp back and rinsing. Leave the shell on.

2. Cut the zucchini into ¾-inch pieces, the eggplant into ½-inch slices and the tomato into ½-inch slices.

3. Mix the kombucha beverage, oil, chili powder, pepper sauce, garlic and salt. Divide the seasoning into two glass dishes or bowls.

4. Place the shrimp in one container and the veggies in the other and let them marinate while you light the barbecue grill and wait for the coals to get hot.

5. Place shrimp on skewers.

6. When the coals are hot, place veggies around the outside edges of the grill, just barely over the coals. Cook for 4 minutes per side, or until seared and somewhat soft.

7. Place the skewered shrimp on the grill in the middle of the coals. Cook for 2 minutes per side.

KOMBUCHA BREAD

The yeasts in the kombucha brew can make bread rise; however, it takes longer than standard bread yeasts. The results are worth it, though: sweet, chewy, warm loaves of bread with a wonderful crunchy crust. Add a little butter to a slice, and you've reached the height of perfection. You can adjust the mix of flour between whole wheat and unbleached white flour to your own taste. However, the kombucha yeasts may have a hard time making the heavier whole wheat rise. This recipe makes 2 loaves of bread.

2 cups kombucha beverage (what works best is to take the liquid and sediment from the bottom of the brewing culture when you're bottling your latest batch)

¼ cup white sugar

¼ cup oil

2 teaspoons salt

6–7 cups flour (any combination of unbleached white and whole wheat)

1. In a large glass bowl, warm the kombucha beverage in the oven set as low as it will go—the mid-80s seems to be ideal.

2. Add sugar, oil and salt. Stir gently. Place the bowl back in the oven for about 10 minutes, until the solution begins to bubble a little.

3. Mix in 4–5 cups of flour until the dough reaches a consistency where it sticks together and you can easily remove it from the bowl.

4. Turn dough onto floured surface and knead about 10 minutes, adding flour as needed. You know

you've kneaded enough and added enough flour when the dough is stretchy and smooth.

5. Place dough in an oiled glass or stainless steel bowl, brush the top with oil, cover with a cloth, and let rise in a warm (about 85°) place until doubled. This may take 2 hours, or even longer.

6. Punch down the dough and divide it in half.

7. On a floured surface, roll out each section of dough into a rectangle.

8. Roll up the dough tightly, starting from the short side. Tuck in the ends under the loaf.

9. Place in oiled bread pans, cover and let rise 1 hour.

10. Bake at 400° for about 35 minutes. The loaves should sound somewhat hollow when done, but they will have a little more moisture in them than your typical bread.

Kombucha for Personal Hygiene

You can even do more with kombucha than using it in your diet. From mouthwash to foot soaks, kombucha has a range of uses for personal hygiene.

If you're going to try using the kombucha brew for personal hygiene, dilute it first: About ¼ cup of the brew to ¾ cup water. Please note that if you plan to apply the brew or the kombucha culture directly to your skin, test a little spot first. The brew and culture are both acidic and might burn sensitive skin.

Mouthwash

Choose a batch of brew that is more acidic than sweet. After all, you wouldn't gargle with sugar-water. Gargle with the diluted brew as you would ordinarily use a mouthwash. Also, drinking the brew first thing in the morning seems to substantially relieve "morning breath." Gargling with the brew may also relieve pain from sore throats or sensitive gums.

Facial Tonic or After-shave

Splash the diluted kombucha brew on your face after shaving or after removing makeup. Also try using the diluted brew as a moisturizer—especially before applying makeup in the morning.

Skin Cream

Buzz an old culture or two in the blender. Add some water until the mixture is at a consistency you can use. Apply to your face as you would normally apply skin cream or a facial mask. Use caution: If you feel a burning sensation, remove the mixture immediately. Sensitive skin may react to the culture's acidity.

Hair Rinse

After shampooing, work about ½ cup of the diluted brew thoroughly into your hair. Let it sit one minute. Rinse out completely. It's supposed to be great for controlling dandruff.

First-aid Rinse

The ingredients in the kombucha brew make it a potent first-aid antiseptic and antibacterial rinse. Apply the diluted brew to the affected area with a cotton ball or gauze pad.

Kombucha Foot Soak

What better way to ease the stress of the day than by soaking your feet in kombucha? Try putting about a cup of the kombucha brew into a gallon of warm, sudsy water. (Always check the water temperature with your elbow first to avoid burning your toes.) Stick your feet in and relax. You may find that corns and calluses soften and that the kombucha soak is a refreshing muscle relaxer.

Try Making Kombucha Extract

If you can't stomach the kombucha brew, but want to reap some of kombucha's benefits, you can try making kombucha extract. The extract is made from the cultures themselves, so it may not have as many nutrients in them as the brew. However, some people claim to have more energy when taking the extract than when drinking the brew. The extract may be better than the beverage for people with diabetes (the cultures have no added sugar in them), for those who don't like the taste of the beverage, or for convenience when traveling. The recommended amount to use ranges from 10 to 25 drops in a glass of water two to three times per day.

EQUIPMENT AND SUPPLIES

    Garlic press or orange juice press

    Muslin cloth

    Small glass container with eyedropper lid

INGREDIENTS

Newer kombucha cultures (not too thick)

Ethyl alcohol (70–90 percent, make sure it's not "denatured," which means it has been made unfit to drink)

STEPS

1. Line the press with muslin cloth.

2. Press the cultures, catching the drops in a glass container.

3. Add an equal amount of ethyl alcohol to the expressed drops. This should give the extract a total alcohol content of about 35 percent.

4. Store the extract in a cool, dark place. The refrigerator should do just fine.

5. Variation: If you can't find ethyl alcohol, try the recipe without it. (Don't use isopropyl rubbing alcohol or "denatured" alcohol, which cannot be digested by your body.) But without the alcohol as a preservative, you'll have to be sure to refrigerate the extract and use it up soon.

Other Uses

Get creative with your kombuchas! Others have. Here are some additional ways you can use the kombucha culture and the beverage.

Around the House

Because the kombucha brew has properties and acids similar to that of vinegar, it makes a helpful household cleaner and solvent. Use about 1 cup of the brew to about 1 gallon of water. Try it on windows (using newspapers and a squeegee works great), greasy areas and anywhere else you would normally use a vinegar solution. Make sure the brew you use for cleaning has fermented long enough to remove most of the sugar, or you may end up with sticky surfaces.

Speaking of sweet sticky surfaces, you may find that the kombucha brew can serve as an inexpensive, nontoxic pesticide. Try coating strips of white or yellow cardboard with undiluted brew. (You may then want to coat the boards with a stickier nontoxic substance such as Tanglefoot.) Place the strips in areas where flies and other garden pests congregate (in fruit trees, in the vegetable garden). I've even used kombucha brew as bug bait. Place the brew in a container set into the ground. Snails, cutworms, sow bugs, ants and who knows what else will gallop toward the sweet, fermented beverage and land in the container, never to rise out again. Every morning, empty the container and refill it with more kombucha brew.

Using Dried Cultures

Believe it or not, there are reports of people drying kombucha cultures and making things out of them: gloves (after tanning the cultures), balloons, even a dried mix that could later be reconstituted with water. I couldn't find any good instructions for these kombucha projects, but if you end up with too many cultures in your brew, give it a try! At the very least, it might make an interesting craft project for your kids.

Some people even propose that the cellulose that covers the kombucha culture is a potentially useful renewable source for both paper and fabric products (such as rayon). Maybe you can be the one to figure out how to do it. With kombucha, the sky is the limit!

8

BUT WHAT ABOUT . . .

Now you've read how the kombucha culture works and how to brew and use the tea, but you're likely to have some additional questions. Here are some common questions that arise, followed by my responses.

Deciding Whether to Try Kombucha

Q: Will kombucha make me healthier?

A: That's a tough question to answer. Many people have reported healthy benefits after using kombucha. But whether or not you use kombucha is a decision only you can make—and only you can take responsibility for. In that sense, it's not any different than any other health decision you make. If you decide to try kombucha, it should simply form a small part of your overall plan to eat and live a full and healthy life, which should include the following steps:

- Eat low-fat, high-fiber foods, including lots of fruits, vegetables and whole grains.

- Drink plenty of water—try for eight glasses a day.

- Get regular exercise.
- Control stress.
- Don't smoke.
- Don't abuse drugs or alcohol.

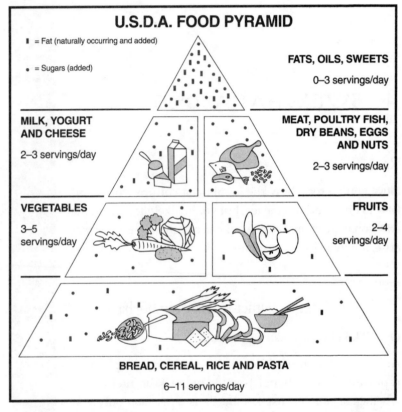

U.S.D.A. FOOD PYRAMID

❚ = Fat (naturally occurring and added)

• = Sugars (added)

FATS, OILS, SWEETS
0–3 servings/day

MILK, YOGURT AND CHEESE
2–3 servings/day

MEAT, POULTRY FISH, DRY BEANS, EGGS AND NUTS
2–3 servings/day

VEGETABLES
3–5 servings/day

FRUITS
2–4 servings/day

BREAD, CEREAL, RICE AND PASTA
6–11 servings/day

Whether or not you decide to use kombucha, following these guidelines is a good way to begin developing healthy eating habits.

Q: I have diabetes. Is it okay to try kombucha?

A: Check with your doctor first. If you decide to try the kombucha beverage, remember that it does contain simple sugars—and the sweeter it tastes, the more sugar it contains. You'll have to account for the extra sugar in your diet just as if you were eating an extra cookie or other sweetened food.

Q: What are some of the possible benefits of drinking the kombucha beverage?

A: Kombucha may have positive effects on your overall well-being. Here are some of the benefits people have noted:

Nutritional Benefits

Many of the consistently identified components of the kombucha brew have well-established nutritional benefits. These include vitamins, minerals and acids that your body needs every day.

Reports of Improved Well-being

Anecdotal reports from thousands of people in all walks of life state that drinking the kombucha beverage has improved their general health and well-being. Many people make even stronger claims that the brew has relieved symptoms of various diseases (see Chapter 4 for more on this). Remember, however, that these claims have not been tested in any recent rigorous scientific study—yet. Most of the studies done in Russia and Germany date from the 1920s to the 1960s.

Psychological Benefits from Taking Charge of Your Health

Taking a positive step to improve your health can have psychological benefits. Rather than falling victim to bad health, you can do something concrete to take charge of your body. You can't help but feel better about yourself. As a result, you may find yourself beginning to make other changes to improve your health.

The Enjoyment of Growing and Sharing Kombucha

It's enjoyable to watch the kombucha culture grow and divide, and then to share the offspring and tea with others. It's the same kind of satisfaction you get from nurturing a garden and watching it thrive because of your care.

Learning about Important Biological Processes

Brewing the tea can be a learning experience for your whole family. Not only do you find out about the processes involved in kombucha fermentation, you can venture into other related foods such as bread, beer, yogurt and vinegar. And it's a short step from learning about kombucha's growth to understanding biological processes such as fermentation and composting. Studying kombucha could even make a great science fair project for school-age children.

Easy to Brew

Once you get the hang of it, brewing kombucha is relatively easy. Starting a new batch takes about an hour, and you can get some other things done (read a magazine, write a letter) while you're waiting for the water to boil and the tea to steep or cool down.

Low Cost

After a possible initial investment in utensils and the kombucha culture, brewing kombucha is inexpensive. All you need is sugar, black tea (Lipton's or any other common brand is fine) and distilled or filtered water.

Relatively Low Chance of Contamination

The greatest danger posed by brewing the kombucha culture is contamination by molds such as *Aspergillus*. However, analyses of the kombucha brew by objective sources have failed to turn up signs of contaminants or other dangerous substances. This may be due to some of the acidic ingredients in the kombucha culture, which may inhibit the development of harmful molds and bacteria.

Q: I've tried kombucha—and I believe it improved my well-being. How can I convince my family and friends to try it, too?

A: Health decisions such as whether or not to try kombucha are very personal. Grant others the same opportunity you had to explore all the options concerning the kombucha beverage. You may believe kombucha will be beneficial for someone but never pressure anyone into drinking it. People need to come to their own conclusions about this exotic beverage. Rather than using strong-arm tactics, simply pass along objective information—such as this book—and let the reader form his or her own opinion.

The Brewing Technique

Q: How do I know if my kombucha culture is okay?

A: There are several things you can do to make certain you have a quality culture. First, be sure you get the culture from a trusted source.

Second, know how the culture was brewed. If black or green tea was used and the instructions in this book were at least roughly followed, the culture is probably okay. If herbal tea was used, don't use the culture. Many herbal teas contain oils that can react with the culture and produce toxic byproducts. If bad brewing techniques were used, keep looking for another source. If the wrong equipment was used, including the container, pass the culture by. One of the few warnings the Food and Drug Administration has issued about kombucha has been in regard to containers. Make sure you don't use a painted, ceramic or leaded crystal container because they all could leach lead into your tea. (If non-lead glazes were used for a ceramic container, it's probably okay.)

Third, as long as the culture keeps fermenting your tea and creating new cultures, it's probably okay. If you see weird colors (green, black or pink) on it, you may have a mold contamination problem. If the mold comes off readily when you rinse the culture with vinegar and cool water, keep the culture, but throw away the batch of tea. Try to brew a new batch with the culture. If you still get signs of contamination, ditch the kombucha and find a new one.

Fourth, if the culture falls apart in your hands when you pick it up, throw it out. A healthy kombucha should be fairly durable—and should at least be able to withstand being picked up and rinsed. If the kombucha readily falls apart, it probably is either too old or contaminated with mold. In either case, throw it out.

Q: How long can I use the "mom"?

A: Use the guidelines in the answer above to determine the quality of the "mom." I've seen recommendations ranging from 5 to 15 times. There are some fears—and possibly some evidence—that the culture begins to mutate the older it gets. Because you're generating new cultures with each batch, there's no reason you can't switch to a new culture fairly frequently.

Q: I see all these little white warts on top of the culture. What are they?

A: As long as they're just clear-looking white warts, your culture is doing just fine. In fact, what you're seeing are air bubbles. As the culture creates new babies on top, air gets trapped between them. In time, the baby and original culture will become more separate.

Q: What do I do with all those extra cultures?

A: You can always give away the extra cultures. If you do so, place a culture in a sealable bag (Ziplocs work great) along with some tea. And ALWAYS pass along instructions with the culture. You'll find an extra copy of the instructions in the back of this book. Or if you really like this person, do him or her a favor and buy them a copy of this book.

Q: How do I dispose of my old kombucha culture?

A: If you need to discard a culture, dispose of it in the trash or bury it outside (try putting it in a compost pile). Don't put it down the drain. There has been some concern that if conditions are right, the culture could continue to grow in your sewer or septic system, creating more employment opportunity for your local plumber.

Q: What do I do if I have to leave town?

A: It's sort of like trying to decide what to do with your pets when you go on vacation, isn't it? If you're only going to be gone a week and a half or less, just start a new batch of tea brewing and it will be ready when you get back. If you plan on being away for a few weeks, keep the culture in a cool place, and you'll have a stronger kombucha vinegar when you return. If you're going to be gone longer than that, you'll have to do some planning. It's probably not reasonable to take the culture with you (although I have taken jars of the brew along in the cooler when I've gone camping). You probably don't have the ability to quick-freeze it, and putting your culture in the freezer is liable to damage it beyond reasonable use. So, here are some alternatives:

- Find a good place to "board" your culture. Hopefully you have a friend or two who you can trust to guard your brew. Be sure to give them complete instructions.

- Place a new batch of fermenting brew, bowl and all, in the refrigerator (keep it covered with the cloth). The cool temperature should suspend most of the culture's activity without killing off the culture itself. Word has it that you can leave the culture in this state of hibernation for up to a few months. When you return, start up a new batch. It may take a couple of batches before your kombucha is back to normal. If the culture hasn't recovered by the end of the third batch, throw it out and get a new culture.

Q: I've heard that it's important for the tea to have the right pH level. What is that? How can I check it?

A: Let's start with defining just what "pH" is. In chemistry, pH means the "potential of hydrogen." Think of it as a scale that starts at 0.1 and

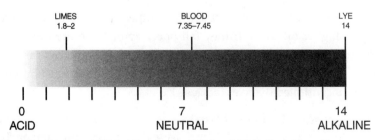

The pH scale starts at 0.1 (acid) and goes as high as 14 (alkaline). The midway point, about 7, is "neutral."

goes as high as 14. What's the midpoint? Approximately 7. We'll call that "neutral." The high point (14) is "alkaline" and the low point (0.1) is "acid."

Our favorite fluid, water, just happens to be neutral. Take a step back to high school science class and remember what water is made up of: H_2O. This formula means that one molecule of water is made up of two hydrogen atoms and one oxygen atom.

When you fill up a glass from your tap and set it down on the counter, the water looks pretty stable. But what you can't see is the ongoing struggle between all those H and O atoms. Some of the molecules break up, leaving extra H atoms and some OH combinations floating around.

When there are more single Hs in the water (or in any other liquid) than there are H_2Os, the liquid is "acid." Acidity measures from 0.1 (very acidic) to 6.9 (slightly acidic) on the pH scale.

When there are more OHs in a liquid than there are H_2Os, liquid is "alkaline." Alkalinity measures from 7.1 (slightly alkaline) to 14 (very alkaline) on the pH scale.

Most substances have a measurable pH level. This includes various areas throughout your body, such as your blood, your urine and your digestive tract. Liquids such as the kombucha beverage also have measurable pH levels.

If you're generally healthy, your pH levels should look like this: Blood has a pH level between 7.35 and 7.45. Saliva is around 7.1. The stomach is very acidic, usually falling between 0.9 and 2.0. Urine is around 6.8.

A bad diet, stress, health problems and other factors can push the pH levels higher or lower. If they fall one way or the other outside the "normal" range, you're likely to become sick. Symptoms can be as mild as a minor stomach upset, or as serious as a life-threatening coma from uncontrolled diabetes (acidosis).

So if you want to find out what some of your pH levels are, you'll have to find a pH testing kit, such as test strips or litmus paper. This may be easier said than done—most drug stores have a hard time putting their hands on pH strips anymore. Pharmacists I've spoken with recommend buying them from a lab supply store or catalog, or finding someone who has access to them in a school chemistry lab. The strips should have instructions for correlating color with pH level. You can try using swimming pool pH testing kits for urine and the kombucha beverage. They're simple to use, although the calibration usually runs only as low as about 6.8 (slightly acidic). But at least you'll have a general idea whether the liquid is acidic or not.

To measure your own pH levels, stick a strip in your mouth first thing in the morning and keep it there for a second or two (*don't use the swimming pool test chemicals for this test*). What's your level? If it's somewhere between 7 and 8, you're in the normal range. The range may be more acidic—that is, less than 7—in children. Check your urine by sticking one of those strips into your urine stream a few seconds after the stream begins. What's the urine level? The reading should be somewhere between 6 and 7.

You can measure the kombucha brew's pH as well, using either the strips or the pool testing kit. There's some debate over what the ideal level of pH for the kombucha brew is. The recommended numbers range anywhere from 2.5 to about 6.0. In any case, it's clear that your kombucha brew should be on the acidic end of the pH scale—that is, below 7.0. If it's alkaline, you've got a problem—probably contamination. Pitch the brew and try again. Rosina Fasching believes that the beverage is best when it measures a pH of 3.0, probably because she wants a more highly fermented beverage for therapeutic purposes. (Remember, it's her uncle, Dr. Sklenar, who advocated using kombucha as therapy for chronic illnesses.) Others recommend less acidic levels, around 4.5 to 6.0.

In either case, how can the acidity of the kombucha beverage help keep your body's pH levels balanced, considering many of them are slightly alkaline? It's thought that several of the acids in the kombucha beverage may in some way "buffer" against certain body processes becoming too acidic or too alkaline. The acids have a slightly diuretic effect, as well. This enables the body to rid itself of accumulated toxins that may be upsetting the pH levels. Finally, the carbon dioxide and carbonic acid in the kombucha brew join with minerals in the body to form bicarbonates (baking soda is the bicarbonate you're probably most familiar with). These alkaline substances circulate in your blood and help to regulate many of your body's processes. All in all, it looks as though an acidic kombucha brew can help you maintain all the various pH levels to keep your body functioning at its best.

Q: Green or black? Does it really matter what kind of tea I use? Why not my favorite herbal blend?

A: Throughout various reports dating as far back as the 1920s, advice about which tea to use has been inconsistent. I'll try to sort it all out here. Let's start with black and green teas. Both come from the same tea plant. But each is processed differently. For green tea, the leaves are picked, steamed, rolled and quickly dried. This process maintains the leaves' green color. For black tea, the leaves are picked, partly dried and rolled. Because they're "crisper" when rolled, the leaves break apart, exposing more of the tea to the air (a fermentation process similar to what the bacteria does in the kombucha culture). As a result, the tea turns brown. When the tea achieves the right color and texture, it is dried with hot air, causing the leaves to turn black.

Black tea is traditionally the tea of choice for brewing kombucha. Black tea contains both caffeine and tannic acid, which apparently help the kombucha culture grow. But because of the additional fermentation process it undergoes, black tea contains higher levels of caffeine and lower levels of tannin than does green tea. Black tea also contains a few antioxidants that may help protect against some cancers. As for its contribution to the taste of the kombucha brew, black tea gives the beverage a fuller, less bitter flavor than green tea will.

Many people do use green tea in their kombucha brews, but usually not exclusively. They generally combine three green tea bags with two black tea bags in three quarts of water. The resulting flavor of the kombucha beverage is slightly more bitter, because of the higher level of tannin in green tea. People who decide to use green tea believe that they're profiting from its health benefits. In fact, green tea does have a proven anticancer effect. It contains antioxidants called "polyphenols" that help protect against cancers of the stomach, colon, skin, lungs and liver.

Oolong tea is similar to black and green teas. The length of the fermentation process for oolong tea falls between black and green teas. Presumably, then, the nutrient, caffeine and tannin content is also somewhere between black and green. If you try oolong, you should still use one or two black tea bags in your brew.

Black, green and oolong teas all come from the same types of tea leaves. The differences in appearance and flavor are due to differences in processing.

The story is much different when it comes to herbal teas, which have countless combinations of hundreds of plants. Many herbal teas are innocuous and simply refreshing. Others can have a powerful, druglike impact on your body. Herbal teas may also contain certain oils that can react with the kombucha culture. The positive effects you notice from drinking herbal teas may be okay when you're sipping an herbal tea to soothe nerves, fall asleep or relieve a stomachache. But the ingredients in many herbal teas can be down-right dangerous to you or at least to the kombucha if the tea is used as the brewing medium.

Advice differs about whether to use herbal teas at all when brewing kombucha. If you really are determined to use herbal tea, you may want to use only milder teas, such as those made up of fruit blossoms (blackberry, raspberry, strawberry or orange, for example). Stronger, medicinal herbs have an ability to destroy or slow down the growth of bacteria, due to their high levels of volatile oils. These oils could probably also damage the bacteria in kombucha. Because of this, I recommend avoiding herbal teas until there has been more complete analysis of their interactions with the kombucha culture. With any type of herbal tea that you might use to brew the culture, you'll probably notice that the fermentation process occurs much more slowly.

In any case, it's up to you to decide which tea to use. As long as you stick to black, green or oolong, you shouldn't have any real trouble.

The safety of herbal teas is less clear. Realize that you are taking more of a chance if you use herbal teas in your brew.

Other Uses for the Culture

Q: Can I give kombucha to my pets? Do I give them the actual fungus?

A: If you decide to use kombucha on a pet, use it sparingly—only a drop or two of extract or a teaspoon or two of the brew in their water dish. Most pets are much smaller than their human companions, so you need to scale back the amount accordingly. There are reports of pets bouncing back from skin diseases after receiving a few drops of the extract. You can also apply diluted brew directly to your pet's skin to relieve itching caused by fleas or allergies.

Q: What about plants? Can they benefit from kombucha?

A: Many sources recommend burying the spent or extra cultures in your garden or compost pile. However, there has been no recent research into whether the particular yeasts and bacteria found in the kombucha culture are beneficial or detrimental to plants. There are, however, some earlier Russian studies that mention improved growth and fewer problems with disease when trees were watered with the brew.

Safety Concerns

Q: What are the risks associated with kombucha?

A: Few side effects have been directly linked to kombucha. However, it is always a good idea to examine all possible risks for anything new that you're considering. Here are some issues to think about:

Imprecise Knowledge about the Kombucha Culture

Although kombucha has existed for thousands of years, it is still not well understood. There remains plenty of disagreement about what's in the brew. Furthermore, there's no complete understanding of all the complex effects of the brew's components on the human body. Of course, this is true of practically every substance you eat or drink. In addition, there have been no recent, widespread scientific studies verifying health claims made about kombucha.

If You Have Weakened Body Defenses

If you have any health condition that weakens your body's defenses, kombucha may do you more harm than good. These conditions include diabetes, HIV, AIDS and possibly conditions such as arthritis. The dilemma is that there are people suffering from these conditions who claim that kombucha has been effective—at least in relieving symptoms. However, kombucha's antibiotic-like tendencies may sometimes backfire in those suffering from these conditions, causing even more health problems. People with these conditions may also be more likely to react to any contaminant in the brew. No one knows for sure. The same is true for the very young and the very old, who are generally more susceptible to toxins and contaminants.

If you have a health condition such as one of those described above, make sure you have a qualified health care practitioner who is willing to monitor your condition while you use kombucha. Start slowly and cautiously to see how kombucha affects you.

If You Have Liver Problems

People with impaired liver function should be careful with kombucha. The liver's role is, among other things, to remove toxins from your body. Additional toxins can be released when you drink the kombucha beverage. If you have a liver problem, these additional toxins could perhaps overwhelm your liver. Also, like people with weakened body defenses, you may be more susceptible to any contaminants that find their way into the beverage.

If You Have Yeast Allergies

If you have yeast allergies, you should probably avoid the kombucha brew. If you think you want to try it anyway, check with your health care provider first. See if your health care provider can help determine which yeasts you are allergic to if you don't already know. They may not be the yeasts commonly found in kombucha, although be aware that other types of yeasts may reside in the culture due to normal variations, mutations or contamination.

If You Are Pregnant or Breastfeeding

If you're pregnant or breastfeeding, it's possible that toxins freed up by the kombucha brew could circulate through the placenta or breast milk to your child—before your liver has a chance to remove them. Since no one knows for sure, it's probably not worth the risk to your baby.

The Necessity of a Careful Brewing Technique

Brewing kombucha tea requires both a careful, clean technique and a few special utensils. It's not difficult, but you do have to pay attention to details. Otherwise, dangerous contaminants can be introduced into the brew.

Unreliable Sources for the Culture

The kombucha culture itself may not be from a reliable source. It's possible for various cultures to have varying components, including dangerous impurities. If the culture wasn't handled properly, the culture and any of its offspring may contain contaminants—even deadly molds.

Q: I've heard that a few people have died from drinking kombucha tea. Is this true?

A: One woman did die. She apparently drank large amounts of the tea, and suffered from many health conditions, including diabetes. That's why you should be very cautious about using the brew if you have any serious condition, especially one like diabetes, which involves the immune system and glucose.

A few other folks have gotten seriously ill from drinking the tea. So far, the illnesses have been traced back to contamination of the tea, probably due to poor brewing habits or starting with a moldy culture. In the case of brewing kombucha tea, cleanliness truly is next to godliness!

Q: I have a serious medical condition, and I'm hoping the kombucha brew will do me some good. Should I try it?

A: Only you can answer that question, and it's a tough one. Some people who have serious medical problems have found the kombucha beverage to be beneficial. But until more is known about the components of the tea and the effects on the body, think twice about drinking the beverage if you have any of the following conditions:

- Diabetes.
- HIV or AIDS.
- Any other condition in which the immune system is weakened.

If you still feel you want to try kombucha, then find a qualified health professional who is willing to monitor your progress. And start slowly.

Q: I'm pregnant. Is it okay to drink the tea?

A: Until more "official" research occurs, don't drink the kombucha beverage if you're pregnant, trying to become pregnant or nursing—and don't give kombucha to young children. There are some concerns (only theories, but still worth noting) that toxins set free by drinking the beverage could circulate through the placenta or breast milk and enter your child. Not a pleasant thought! And kombucha is not recommended for young children because their bodies are already running in such high gear. Giving them the kombucha brew may be overdoing it. If you are pregnant and insist on trying kombucha anyway, be sure you're being monitored by a qualified health professional.

Q: But isn't this just another New Age "alternative medicine" fad?

A: As time passes, the differences between "alternative" and "traditional" medicine are fading. The broad interest in kombucha reinforces this trend. Many "traditional" physicians take the kombucha culture and beverage seriously, as do many research scientists. Rather than immediately writing off the potential benefits from the kombucha culture and its brew, most scientists involved in health and nutrition, including the FDA, are taking more of a "wait and see" attitude: They are cautious and tentative and don't automatically disclaim any potential benefits. Most alternative health practitioners take a cautiously positive approach to kombucha. In any case, it's important to have health care professionals as part of your "team" who will work with you in a variety of ways—with or without kombucha—to improve and maintain your good health.

Q: So just who is this "qualified health professional" I should work with?

A: There really are medical doctors out there who are open to working with patients who want to try "alternative" health remedies. Ask around at your local health food store to get names. Don't be afraid to follow up with a call to someone you see quoted in a magazine, newspaper article or TV report.

You can also consider adding a new member to your health care team—a licensed naturopath, herbalist or nutritionist who has experience with kombucha. But whatever you do, don't become part of this *Consumer Reports* statistic: They estimate that 72 percent of the people who use some sort of alternative medicine treatment don't tell their regular medical doctors about it. This is only setting yourself up for potential trouble. All too often one health care practitioner recommends something that may conflict with what another health care practitioner is prescribing. Prescription drugs and herbal interactions are just one possible example. So be sure to let all members of your health care team know who you're working with and what medications and therapies you're taking, including substances such as kombucha. That way you can be sure your health care is more coordinated—and that you're doing as much good for yourself as possible.

But what if some of your health care providers scoff at you? You're tough enough to take it. Give them all the information you can about what you're considering doing and keep everyone posted on your progress.

CONCLUSION

When I first learned of kombucha, I was immediately in-
trigued by its use in Eastern Europe. After all, my ancestors
came from that part of the world. How perfect it would be
if someone remembered that Great-grandmother Tarsenko
kept a kombucha brewing in the corner of her kitchen in
Hamtramck (an Eastern European enclave in Detroit). Or
maybe that Grandpa Petro carried a flask of the beverage
with him on his long, frightening journey from Russia to
Canada in 1917.

Unfortunately, it seems that none of my relatives were
involved in the tradition of brewing kombucha. Nevertheless, studying kombucha's history and uses has been an
enjoyable journey for me. Not only has it given me knowledge about an unusual and fascinating substance. It has
also helped me to understand more about life processes
such as fermentation that are all around us, but that are
usually taken for granted. It has encouraged me to be more
observant about my own health on a day-to-day basis. And
it has given me a chance to experience first-hand the benefits from brewing and drinking the kombucha beverage.

You, too, have now traveled around the world with this exotic "Tea Mushroom." You've learned about the lore surrounding kombucha, about the components of the fungus, about brewing and using it. You may decide to try brewing kombucha yourself. If you do, keep this book handy for a quick reference. If you decide not to try kombucha, at least take to heart the underlying kombucha message: Strive to do all you can to live a healthy and satisfying life, no matter what your age or what your health status may be. I hope this journey has been—and will continue to be—a worthwhile adventure for you.

GLOSSARY

ACETATE. A group of solvent-like substances that can form when acetic acid sits around too long and reacts with other substances such as alcohol or cellulose.

ACETOBACTER ACETI. One of the three known groups of bacteria identified in the kombucha culture.

ACETOBACTER ACETI SUBSPECIES XYLINUM (BROWN) COMB. NOV. One of the three known groups of bacteria identified in the kombucha culture. Apparently, it has also gone by the name of *Acetobacter ketogenum.* (People once believed they were two different bacteria.)

ACID. A substance that ranges from 0.1 to 6.9 on the pH scale. Several types of acids are used for many purposes in your body, including building proteins.

AEROBE. Meaning "with air." Aerobe is used to describe bacteria that need oxygen in order to generate energy. The bacteria in the kombucha culture are aerobic bacteria.

ALCOHOL. A very simple carbohydrate that requires little digestion.

ALKALINE. A substance measuring above 7.0 on the pH scale.

AMINO ACID. A "building block" for protein.

ANAEROBE. Meaning "without air."

ANTIOXIDANT. A sort of natural preservative. Antioxidants help keep the body functioning properly by preventing toxic substances from causing damage.

ASCORBIC ACID. Another term for vitamin C.

ASPERGILLUS. A mold that appears on food. If eaten, aspergillus can cause illness (food poisoning) and even death.

BACTERIA. One-celled organisms that rely on organic matter for their food source.

BICARBONATE. A substance that's made up of carbon, oxygen and a mineral (either sodium, potassium, calcium or magnesium). The bicarbonates found in your blood keep your blood slightly alkaline, its preferred pH range.

BUDDING. One way that yeasts reproduce. The other two ways are through spores (like mushrooms) and cell division. The yeasts in the kombucha culture all reproduce through budding.

CAFFEINE. A bitter white substance that serves as a mild stimulant and leads to weight loss. Caffeine enables the kombucha brewing process.

CARBON DIOXIDE. This gas, chemically called CO_2, is given off during the kombucha brewing process. When mixed with water, it turns into carbonic acid.

CARBONIC ACID. An acid created when carbon dioxide mixes with water in the kombucha brew. The result? Fizziness.

CELLULOSE. A type of very complex carbohydrate found in the cell walls of most plants and animals, including your own body.

CHA. The Japanese word for "tea."

COMPOSTING. A process by which organic (formerly living) material is broken down into simpler components.

CULTURE. A group of microorganisms that grow in a specific environment or medium.

DETOXIFICATION. The process by which the liver removes dangerous substances from your body.

DIURETIC. Any substance that causes the body to lose fluid.

ENZYME. A substance that is able to help cells generate energy without being used up itself.

ERGOSTEROL. A waxy substance found in yeast and used by your body to generate vitamin D.

ETHANOL. A type of alcohol. Ethanol is found in beer, wine, sake and other alcoholic beverages.

FERMENTATION. The process by which more complex sugars are converted by yeasts into simpler sugars, and ultimately to alcohol. It's the first step of the kombucha brewing process.

FUNGUS JAPONICUS. The pharmaceutical name for the kombucha culture.

GLUCONIC ACID. An acid created by one of the bacteria in the kombucha culture. It may have some preservative value in the kombucha beverage.

GLUCONOBACTER OXYDANS SUBSPECIES SUBOXYDANS (KLUYVER AND DE LEEUW) COMB. NOV. One of the three known groups of bacteria identified in the kombucha culture. It has also been called *Bacterium gluconicum.*

HERBALIST. A health care practitioner who has training or experience in prescribing herbs for specific health conditions.

IMMUNE SYSTEM. Your body's mechanism for defending against infection and disease.

INVERTASE. An enzyme found in yeasts that helps them break down sugars.

IRON. A mineral that helps carry oxygen in your blood and body tissues.

KLOEKERA APICULATA. One of the four known yeasts identified in the kombucha culture.

KOMBU. The Japanese word for "seaweed." This word has created great confusion in understanding the origins of the word "kombucha," even leading some to assume that the culture was originally brewed in some sort of seaweed tea or that the Japanese thought the culture was a sort of seaweed.

LACTIC ACID. One of the acids left over by the kombucha brewing process. Often used as a food preservative, lactic acid helps deter the growth of harmful bacteria. It may also help encourage the growth of beneficial bacteria in your digestive tract.

MALONIC (MALIC) ACID. One of the acids found in the finished kombucha beverage.

MEDIUM. The environment in which a culture resides. The kombucha culture, for example, needs the medium of sweet black tea. Otherwise, it would starve to death.

MOLD. A type of fungus that is made up of thread-like, cottony substances.

MOTHER. Refers to your original kombucha culture, from which all new kombucha cultures spring forth.

NATUROPATH. A health practitioner who uses natural remedies and therapies for treating health problems and has completed a course of study at a school of naturopathy.

NEUTRAL. Being neither acidic nor alkaline but exactly 7 on the pH scale.

NIACIN. Vitamin B_3, also called nicotinic acid. This vitamin keeps your blood vessels open, regulates your cholesterol levels, helps your nerves work properly and helps create hormones.

NITROGEN. This chemical substance is a component of black tea and acts as a catalyst to help the anaerobic bacteria digest the alcohol and sugars in the tea.

NUTRITIONIST. A general term referring to health care practitioners who give advice about nutrition. Many nutritionists have a master's degree in nutrition and are also registered dietitians (RDs). Some nutritionists focus on traditional diets. "Alternative" nutritionists also use herbs and other substances, such as the kombucha beverage, in their diet prescriptions.

OXALIC ACID. An acid left in the kombucha beverage as a result of the bacteria's action. It may have a slightly diuretic effect on the body, thereby helping to flush out toxins.

PANGAMIC ACID. Vitamin B_{15}. Found in yeast, this vitamin helps your blood carry oxygen.

PANTOTHENIC ACID. Vitamin B_5. Found in yeasts, this vitamin is involved in almost every process your body undertakes. It may also help reduce gray hair.

PARA-AMINO BENZOIC ACID (PABA). This B vitamin absorbs the sun's ultraviolet rays, helps your body produce folic acid and helps prevent gray hair.

PASTEURIZATION. A process whereby a beverage or other food is heated to kill off microorganisms that would otherwise cause the food to spoil. Pasteurization can also kill off beneficial bacteria and yeasts, such as those in the kombucha beverage. However, some nutrients will remain.

PH. The measure of the acidity or alkalinity of a liquid on a scale of 0 to 14. The midpoint of the scale is 7: neutral. Above 7 means the solution is alkaline and below 7 means the solution is acidic.

PHOSPHORUS. A mineral found in the kombucha beverage that, along with calcium, helps your body make and maintain bones.

PICHIA FERMENTANS. One of the four known yeasts identified in the kombucha culture.

POLYPHENOLS. Antioxidant substances found in green tea that have been shown to protect against stomach, colon, skin, lung and liver cancers. Black tea may also contain these substances, though to a lesser extent.

POTASSIUM. A mineral that, like sodium, is found in your body's fluids. It helps regulate body fluids, muscle contractions, nerve function, protein formation, glucose breakdown and heart rhythm.

PYRIDOXINE. Vitamin B_6. Found in yeasts, this vitamin helps you digest and use proteins and fats, regulates body fluids, lowers your risk of artery disease, relieves symptoms of depression and helps maintain healthy skin and your body's immune system. Most people get only about half of what they should of this critical vitamin.

RIBOFLAVIN. Vitamin B_2. Found in yeasts, this vitamin helps your body break down fats, use oxygen, lessen the symptoms of depression and prevent cataracts.

SACCHAROMYCODES LUDWIGII. One of the four known yeasts identified in the kombucha culture.

SALMONELLA. In the early 1900s David E. Salmon discovered this type of bacteria, which is responsible for most cases of food poisoning.

SCHIZOSACCHAROMYCES POMBE. One of the four known yeasts identified in the kombucha culture.

SCURVY. A disease resulting from a vitamin C deficiency.

STAPHYLOCOCCUS AUREUS. A common but undesirable type of bacteria that is responsible for a range of ills, including skin infections, toxic shock syndrome, bone infection and food poisoning from dairy and meat products.

SUCCINIC ACID. Found in the finished kombucha beverage, this acid probably has some preservative effect on the brew and a detoxifying effect on your body.

SUCROSE. A carbohydrate made up of two separate sugars: glucose and fructose. It's the major component of white sugar and the sugar of choice for brewing the kombucha beverage.

SULFUR. One of the minerals needed by your body, sulfur is found in the proteins of your hair, nails and cartilage and helps rid your body of toxic substances.

TANNIN (TANNIC ACID). Used to tan hides, this acid is also in black and green tea. (Depending on the amount in the tea, it can make the tea taste bitter.)

TARTARIC ACID. Found in the finished kombucha beverage, this acid probably has some preservative effect on the brew and a detoxifying effect on your body.

TEA KVASS. The Russian term for the kombucha beverage. (Kvass is a weak Russian beer made from black bread, water and sugar. The brewing technique and end result resemble the kombucha brew.)

TOXIN. Any substance that can damage your body. Toxins can be metals, chemicals, organisms and other substances.

ULTRAVIOLET (UV) LIGHT. A type of invisible radiation generated by sunlight, UV rays can be damaging to the kombucha culture.

USNIC ACID. An antibacterial substance found in some lichens, which may also prevent tumors from growing.

VOLATILE OILS. Found in many of the plants used in herbal teas, these oils can damage the bacteria in the kombucha culture.

YEAST. A type of fungus.

ON-LINE RESOURCES

If you just can't seem to get enough information about kombucha, don't worry. If you know where to look, you can find lots more about your favorite fungal culture. In the bibliography, I've listed the print sources that were helpful to me in researching this book. Especially fascinating, though, is the information that's available on the internet through the on-line services and governmental agencies. If you've been computer-shy in the past, maybe now's the time to learn how to "surf" the "net" for kombucha information. Following are some suggestions to help you get started.

Computer-based Resources

If you have a computer and modem, the only other thing you need is a service that will allow you to use the internet. The on-line commercial services all provide internet access, although their ease of use varies greatly. You can also sign up with several other companies that specialize in providing internet services.

Many times, all you'll want to do on the internet is have discussions with people who share your interests or are doing research. You may also want to find some relevant pages on the world wide web (WWW). This part of the internet is made up of thousands of "home pages" that provide information (often about commercial products and services) and offer links to similar sources of information.

In all cases, you need to realize that the internet is an unpoliced system. There's no one who documents or verifies that any of the information on the internet is reliable. But if you track down a magazine article on the internet, it's as credible as if it were printed on paper and bound, even though it probably has a few typos and may be missing some graphics. Forum discussions and WWW pages are different. Forums have systems operators (sysops) who keep everything up and running and chide people when they're getting too obnoxious. But they have no authority to do anything more than post information that has been submitted by forum participants. Many WWW home pages are developed either by a company with an agenda (to sell a product) or by someone as a hobby. Because much of the information on home pages is presented in a sophisticated graphic style, it's tempting to assume that it must be true. Always remember to read everything with some skepticism.

If you're interested in learning more about kombucha on-line, check out the following possibilities.

Commercial On-line Services

The three largest commercial on-line services all offer extensive forums, health references and access to many other research databases.

AMERICA ONLINE For information about kombucha, check out the Longevity Forum. There's a Kombucha Tea Mushroom Message Board in the Alternative Medicine section of the forum.

COMPUSERVE You can find information about kombucha in three places: 1) the New Age Forum B, Alternative Health library, 2) the Natural Medicine/Holistic Health Forum (GO:HOLISTIC), several libraries and message boards and 3) the Gardening Forum, Herbs library.

PRODIGY Look for the Health Bulletin Board and then access the Holistic Medicine topic area, specific subject of "kombucha."

World Wide Web Pages

Here are two addresses for a world wide web page that features information on kombucha:

http://www.webcom.com/~sease/kombucha/kombucha.html
http://www.webcom.com/~sease/kombucha/roche.html

You can also find information about kombucha and many other health topics through "Yahoo," a home page that serves as an index to health and alternative health information. Here's the address for Yahoo:

http://www.yahoo.com/

The Kombucha Tea Cider gopher is sponsored by Arizona State University. A "gopher" is software that "tunnels" through all the layers of the internet to find things for you. The internet address for the Kombucha Tea Cider gopher is:

enuxsa.eas.asu.edu 6600

BIBLIOGRAPHY

The following books, articles and other publications proved to be helpful or at least interesting throughout the development of this book.

Academic American Encyclopedia, on-line edition. Grolier, Inc., 1994.

Adams, Ruth. "Antioxidant Vitamins Take Aim at America's Worst Serial Killer: Cardiovascular Disease. C, E and Beta-Carotene Fight Damaging Free Radicals, Regulate Cholesterol." *Health News & Review*, Wntr. 1993, vol. 3, no. 1, p. 22.

"Alternative Medicine: What to Look For." *Consumer Reports*, Jan. 1994.

Anderson, Ronald. "Vitamin C and Immunity." *Nutrition & Food Science*, Sept.–Oct. 1993, no. 5, p. 29.

"The Anticancer Fiber: Insoluble Fiber in Wheat Bran." *The University of California, Berkeley Wellness Letter*, Dec. 1989, vol. 6. no. 3, p. 2.

Arnot, Bob. "Health Check: The Truth About 'Mushroom Tea.' " *Good Housekeeping*, Aug. 1995, p. 56.

"Ascorbic Acid." *USP DI-Volume II Advice for the Patient: Drug Information in Lay Language,* Edition 15, 1995, p. 344.

Austin, Steve and Cathy Hitchcock. "The Linus Pauling–Mayo Clinic Controversy Involving Vitamin C and Cancer Tests." *Nutrition Health Review,* Wntr. 1995, no. 71, p. 10.

"B Makes the Grade." *Consumer Reports on Health,* June 1995, vol. 7, no. 6, p. 61.

"B Vitamin Group Seen Lacking in Diet." *Executive Health's Good Health Report,* Feb. 1994, vol. 30, no. 5, p. 1.

Baker, Elizabeth. "Kombucha: The Fungus Tea." *Total Health,* April 1995, vol. 17, no. 2, p. 42.

Baringa, Marcia. "Vitamin C Gets a Little Respect." *Science,* Oct. 18, 1991, vol. 254, no. 5030, p. 374.

Bentley, J. Peter; Hunt, Thomas K.; Weiss, Jacqueline B.; Taylor, Christopher M.; Hanson, Albert N.; Davies, Gordon H.; Halliday, Betty J. "Peptides from Live Yeast Cell Derivative Stimulate Wound Healing." *Archives of Surgery,* May 1990, vol. 125, no. 5, p. 641.

Berkowitz, Kathy Feld. "Trio of Vitamins Are Recruited in the Fight Against Heart Disease." *Environmental Nutrition,* Sept. 1992, vol. 15, no. 9, p. 1.

Berlin, Linda. "At the Nation's Table: Glob, Glob, Gulp, Gulp." *The New York Times,* Dec. 21, 1994, p. C8.

Bertelsmann Lexikon. Bertelsmann Electronic Publishing, Munich, Germany, 1994.

Bone, James. "America Hails New Miracle Cure-all: Kombucha." *London Times,* Feb. 9, 1995.

Booe, Martin. "Tea Tempest: Is Kombucha a Wonder Drug or Just a Fungus?" *Chicago Tribune,* 1995.

Buchanan, Caroline. "Lecithin Supplements: A Source of Help or Hype?" *Environmental Nutrition,* June 1989, vol. 12, no. 6, p. 1.

"Can Vitamin C Save Your Life?" *Consumer Reports on Health*, March 1994, vol. 6, no. 3, p. 25.

"Caution with Kombucha: Tea with Health Claims Should Not Be Served in Containers with Lead Due to Health Hazard." *FDA Consumer*, June 1995, vol. 29, no. 5, p. 4.

Christen, William Gerard, Jr. "Antioxidants and Eye Disease." *American Journal of Medicine*, Sept. 26, 1994, vol. 97, no. 3A, p. 14S.

"Death and Illness Linked to Kombucha Fad" (Adapted from the *Des Moines Register*, April 13, 1995). *NCAHF Newsletter*, May–June 1995, vol. 18, no. 3, p. 1.

"Diet and Vitamins May Prevent Heart Attack, Stroke." *Aging*, Fall 1994, no. 366, p. 3.

Drake, Geoff. "The Lactate Shuttle: Contrary to What You've Heard, Lactic Acid Is Your Friend." *Bicycling*, August, 1992, vol. 33, no. 7, p. 36.

Fasching, Rosina. *Tea Fungus Kombucha: The Natural Remedy and Its Significance in Cases of Cancer and Other Metabolic Diseases*. Ennsthaler Publishing House, Steyr, Austria, 7th edition, 1995.

"FDA Is Urged to Support the Use of Antioxidants." *Better Nutrition for Today's Living*, July 1994, vol. 56, no. 7, p. 12.

"For Your Heart's Sake: More B Vitamins." *Tufts University Diet & Nutrition Letter*, Feb. 1994, vol. 11, no. 12, p. 1.

Foster, R. Daniel. "Kombucha: Mushroom with a Mission." *Natural Health*, March–April 1995, vol. 25, no. 2, p. 52.

Foster, R. Daniel. "The Mushroom that Ate L.A." *Los Angeles Magazine*, Nov. 1994, p. 118.

Frank, Günther W. *Kombucha: Healthy Beverage and Natural Remedy from the Far East—Its Correct Preparation and Use*. Ennsthaler Publishing House, Steyr, Austria, 7th edition, 1995.

Frei, Balz. "Reactive Oxygen Species and Antioxidant Vitamins: Mechanisms of Action." *American Journal of Medicine*, Sept. 26, 1994, vol. 97, no. 3A, p. 5S.

Gaziano, J. Michael. "Antioxidant Vitamins and Coronary Artery Disease Risk." *American Journal of Medicine*, Sept. 26, 1994, vol. 97, no. 3A, p. 18S.

Gordon, Jeff. "Kombucha: Care and Feeding." CompuServe Holistic Health Forum Library, 1995.

Gruning, Carl. "Seeing Is Believing! For Lifelong Eye Health, Just Remember Your ABCs and these Minerals (Preventing Cataracts, Poor Vision and Glaucoma with Good Nutrition)." *Health News & Review*, Summer 1992, vol. 2, no. 3, p. 1.

Gutfeld, Greg; Sangiorgio, Mauree; Rao, Linda. "Gene Protection: Vitamin C." *Prevention*, July 1992, vol. 44, no. 7, p. 14.

Gutfeld, Greg; Rao, Linda; Sangiorgio, Maureen. "A More Fruitful Life: Vitamin C Linked to Longevity." *Prevention*, Sept. 1992, vol. 44, no. 9, p. 9.

Halliwell, Barry. "Free Radicals, Antioxidants, and Human Disease: Curiosity, Cause, or Consequence?" *The Lancet*, Sept. 10, 1994, vol. 344, no. 8924, p. 721.

Hearn, Wayne. "Mushroom Tea: Toxicity Concerns about New 'Cure-all.' " *American Medical News*, May 1, 1995, vol. 38, no. 17, p. 21.

Hennekens, Charles H. "Antioxidant Vitamins and Cancer." *American Journal of Medicine*, Sept. 26, 1994, vol. 97, no. 3A, p. 2S.

"Heroic Doses: Questionable Benefits of Vitamins C and E as Antioxidants." *The Economist*, August 27, 1994, vol. 332, no. 7878, p. 74.

Heseker, H.; Schneider, R. "Requirement and Supply of Vitamin C, E and Beta-Carotene for Elderly Men and Women." *European Journal of Clinical Nutrition*, Feb. 1994, vol. 48, no. 2, p. 118.

"High C—Sounding Better? Vitamin C Intake and Decreased Mortality." *Harvard Health Letter*, Sept. 1992, vol. 17, no. 11, p. 8.

Hobbs, Christopher. *Kombucha-Manchurian Tea Mushroom: The Essential Guide*. Botanica Press, Santa Cruz, 1995.

Hunter, Beatrice Trum. "An Unsafe Medicinal Tea?" *Consumers' Research Magazine*, August 1995, vol. 78, no. 8, p. 8.

Hunter, David J.; Manson, JoAnn E.; Colditz, Graham A.; Stampfer, Meir J.; Rosner, Bernard; Hennekens, Charles H.; Speizer, Frank E.; Willett, Walter C. "A Prospective Study of the Intake of Vitamins C, E, and A and the Risk of Breast Cancer." *The New England Journal of Medicine*, July 22, 1993, vol. 329, no. 4, p. 234.

Husten, Larry. "Second Thoughts About Antioxidants." *Harvard Health Letter*, Feb. 1995, vol. 20, no. 4, p. 4.

Information Please Almanac, electronic edition. Houghton Mifflin Company, 1995.

"The Japanese Preference for Green Tea." Associated Press Wire Service (AP Online), Nov. 10, 1988.

"The Juice Truth: Beyond Vitamin C." *Environmental Nutrition*, Dec. 1994, vol. 17, no. 12, p. 7.

Kaiser, Chris A.; Preuss, Daphne; Grisafi, Paula; Botstein, David. "Many Random Sequences Functionally Replace the Secretion Signal Sequence of Yeast Invertase." *Science*, Jan. 16, 1987, vol. 235, p. 312.

Kiester, Edwin Jr. *New Family Medical Guide*. Better Homes and Gardens Books, Des Moines, Iowa, 1984.

Kolor, Agnes. "Vitamin C Promises to Fight Cancer as Well as Runny Noses." *Environmental Nutrition*, May 1992, vol. 15, no. 5, p. 1.

"Kombucha Is a Beverage with Many Applications." *Better Nutrition for Today's Living*, July 1995, vol. 57, no. 7, p. 12.

Langer, Stephen. "Antioxidants: Fighting for Your Life." *Better Nutrition for Today's Living*, July 1994, vol. 56, no. 7, p. 38.

Liversidge, Anthony. "Heresy! Three Modern Galileos: Scientific Theories of Linus Pauling, Peter Duesberg, Thomas Gold." *Omni*, June 1993, vol. 15, no. 8, p. 43.

Long, Patricia. "The Power of Vitamin C." *Health*, Oct. 1992, vol. 6, no. 6, p. 66.

"Magnesium, B Vitamins Benefit CFS Patients." *Better Nutrition for Today's Living*, Nov. 1994, vol. 56, no. 11, p. 18.

Martini, Margaret C; Lerebours, Eric C.; Lin, Wei-Jin; Harlander, Susan K.; Berrada, Nabil M.; Antoine, Jean M.; Savaiano, Dennis A. "Strains and Species of Lactic Acid Bacteria in Fermented Milks (Yogurts): Effect on In Vivo Lactose Digestion." *American Journal of Clinical Nutrition*, Dec. 1991, vol. 54, no. 6.

Marwick, Charles. "Cancer Institute Takes a Look at Ascorbic Acid." *The Journal of the American Medical Association*, Oct. 17, 1990, vol. 264, no. 15, p. 1926.

Meehan, Beth Ann. "Linus Pauling's Rehab: New Study Agrees on Benefits of Megadoses of Vitamin C." *Discover*, Jan. 1993, vol. 14, no. 1, p. 54.

Miller, Frederick W. "Unanswered Questions: Health Risks of Sunscreens Containing Octyl Dimethyl PABA." *Allured Publishing Corp.*, June 1989, vol. 104, no. 6, p. 7.

Munson, Marty. "Ducking Damage: Can Vitamin C Stem Diabetic Complications?" *Prevention*, March 1995, vol. 47, no. 3, p. 34.

"A New Reason to B: Vitamin B in Preventing Heart Disease." *Harvard Health Letter*, May 1994, vol. 19, no. 7, p. 1.

O'Neill, Molly. "A Magic Mushroom or a Toxic Fad?" *The New York Times*, Dec. 28, 1994, p. C1.

"Our Vitamin Prescription: The Big Four." *The University of California, Berkeley Wellness Letter*, Jan. 1994, vol. 10, no. 4, p. 1.

Pascal, Alana and Lynne Van der Kar. *Kombucha: How-To and What It's All About*. The Van der Kar Press, Malibu, 1995.

Petrova, Nina. *The Best of Russian Cooking: Recipes from Russia and the Ukraine*. Crown Publishers Inc., New York, 1979.

Pauling, Linus. "The Absolute Latest on Vitamin C from Its Foremost Advocate at 92." *Health News & Review*, Spring 1993, vol. 3, no. 2, p. 8.

Pryor, Betsy and Sanford Holst. *Kombucha Phenomenon: The Health Drink Sweeping America*. Sierra Sunrise Books, Sherman Oaks, CA, 1994.

Rath, Matthias; Pauling, Linus. "Disease and Vitamin C: An Extract from 'A Unified Theory of Human Cardiovascular Disease.' " *Nutrition Health Review*, Spring 1992, no. 62, p. 6.

Rieger, Martin. "Skin Constituents as Cosmetics Ingredients." *Cosmetics and Toiletries*, Nov. 1992, vol. 107, no. 11, p. 85.

Roufs, James. " 'C' How Much Longer You Can Live: New Study Reveals Vitamin C Can Help Prolong Life." *Muscle & Fitness*, Oct. 1992, vol. 53, no. 10, p. 52.

Roufs, James. "Cholesterol & Vitamin C." *Muscle & Fitness*, May 1992, vol. 53, no. 5, p. 50.

Roufs, James. "Cure for the Common Cold?" *Muscle & Fitness*, Nov. 1992, vol. 53, no. 11, p. 54.

Roussin, Michael. "Common Sense Questions for the Lay-Person on the Topic of Kombucha or Manchurian Mushroom Tea." In the CompuServe Holistic Health Forum Library, 1995.

Scheer, James F. "Restating Praise for Dietary Role of Vitamin C." *Better Nutrition for Today's Living*, Feb. 1994, vol. 56, no. 2, p. 22.

Scheer, James F. "The 'Sunshine Supplement' Boosts Your Bone Health: Vitamin D Ensures Absorption of Calcium and Phosphorous from the Intestinal Tract and Transports Them to Key Areas." *Today's Living*, Jan. 1990, vol. 21, no. 1, p. 14.

Scheer, James F. "Vitamin C Learns Some New Tricks." *Better Nutrition for Today's Living*, Feb. 1992, vol. 54, no. 2, p. 18.

"Seldom-Reported Research Around the World: Documenting Important Discoveries in Vitamin C Therapy." *Nutrition Health Review*, Spring 1992, no. 62, p. 6.

Siegler, Bonnie. "Spoiling Herself Healthy." *Longevity Magazine*, May 1995.

Skerrett, P. J.; Zittell, Nicholas K. "Mighty Vitamins: The One-A-Day Wonders Bidding to Outstrip Their Role as Supplements." *Medical World News*, Jan. 1993, vol. 34, no. 1, p. 24.

Solzhenitsyn, Aleksandr I. *The Cancer Ward*. The Dial Press, Inc., New York, 1968.

Szent-Gyorgyi, Albert. "Reflections on Vitamin C and Hidden Scurvy." *Nutrition Health Review*, Spring 1992, no. 62, p. 5.

Treem, William R.; Ahsan, Naheedt; Sullivan, Barbara; Rossi, Thomas; Holmes, Ronald; Fitzgerald, Joseph; Proujansky, Roy; Hyams, Jeffrey. "Limentary Tract: Evaluation of Liquid Yeast-Derived Sucrase Enzyme Replacement in Patients with Sucrase-Isomaltase Deficiency." *Gastroenterology*. Oct. 1993, vol. 10, no. 4, p. 1061.

"USDA Research (Sections on Vitamin D and B12, Chromium, Stearic Acid)." *Nutrition Today*, Feb. 1992, vol. 27, no. 1, p. 5. "Vinegar: No Miracle Cure, But a Handy Condiment to Have Around." *Environmental Nutrition*, May 1994, vol. 17, no. 5, p. 7.

"Vinegar Virtues." *The University of California, Berkeley Wellness Letter*, Aug. 1994, vol. 10, no. 11, p. 2.

"Vitamin B Helps Overcome Depression." *Executive Health's Good Health Report*, Feb. 1993, vol. 29, no. 5, p. 8.

"Vitamin C and Blood Pressure." *Nutrition Research Newsletter*, March 1993, vol. 12, no. 3, p. 28.

"Vitamin C and Colds Revisited" (adapted from the *Journal of the American College of Nutrition*, April 1995). *Nutrition Research Newsletter*, April 1995, vol. 14, no. 4, p. 52.

"Vitamin C and Zinc Aid Infertile Men." *Better Nutrition for Today's Living*, June 1994, vol. 56, no. 6, p. 22.

"Vitamin C (Ascorbic Acid): Good Sources of Nutrients." U.S. Department of Agriculture, Jan. 1990.

"Vitamin C, Fiber May Prevent Breast Cancer." *Better Nutrition for Today's Living*, Dec. 1993, vol. 55, no. 12, p. 16.

"Vitamin C in Respiratory Infections." *Nutrition Research Newsletter*, Jan. 1995, vol. 14, no. 1, p. 10.

"Vitamin C Lowers Risk of Cardiovascular Disease." *Better Nutrition for Today's Living*, Jan. 1995, vol. 57, no. 1, p. 28.

"Vitamin C May Prevent Numerous Cribdeaths." *Better Nutrition for Today's Living*, March 1995, vol. 57, no. 3, p. 42.

"Vitamin C Reported to Prevent Sperm Damage." *Nutrition Health Review*, Spring 1992, no. 62, p. 4.

"Vitamin C: The Secret to a Long Life and a Healthy Heart?" *Environmental Nutrition*, July 1992, vol. 15, no. 7, p. 3.

Weininger, Jean. "Steeped in Tradition, Are Green Teas a Panacea or Just a Pot of Comfort?" *San Francisco Chronicle*, May 10, 1995.

"Will Fiber Save Your Life?" *Consumer Reports Health Letter*, March 1990, vol. 2, no. 3, p. 17.

"Yeast Is Yeast." *The University of California, Berkeley Wellness Letter*, Dec. 1989, vol. 6, no. 3, p. 7.

"Yeast May Help Stop Cancer from Spreading." *Cancer Weekly*, April 19, 1993, p 4.

"Yeast Meets West." *People Weekly*, Feb. 13, 1995, vol. 43, no. 6, p. 192.

INDEX

Plants, 116
PMS, 36
Polyphenols, 114–15
Potassium, 53
Pregnancy, 50, 118, 119
Pronatura (mail-order supplier), 59, 60, 63
Pryor, Betsy, 19, 33
Psoriasis, 34
Psychological benefits, 33, 107
Pyridoxine, 48–49

Qualified health professionals, 120

Rashes, 37
Reagan, Ronald, 20
Recipes, 94–100
Riboflavin, 48
Russia, 11–14, 15

Saccharomycodes ludwigii, 24
Safety concerns, 116–20
Salmonella, 27, 40
Schizosaccharomyces pombe, 24
Scurvy, 42
Search for Health magazine, 18
Serine, 28
Sharing kombucha, 61, 107–108, 110
Side effects, 35, 37–38
Skin, 34, 44, 49
Skin cream, 101
Sklenar, Rudolf, 15–16, 113
Sodium, 53
Solzhenitsyn, Aleksandr, 13, 20
South Africa, 20
Soviet Union (former), 11–14
Spain, 15, 17
Sperm, 43–44
Spicy grilled kombucha shrimp and veggies, 98
Stalin, Joseph, 12–13
Staphylococcus aureus, 40
Starter liquid, 71, 78
Sterols, 4
Storage containers, 84–85, 109
Succinic acid, 29
Sucrase, 51
Sucrose, 23, 24, 26–27
Sudden infant death syndrome (SIDS), 54
Sugar, 23–24, 26–27, 71
Sugar substitutes, 71
Sugars, 51
Sulfur, 53

Supplies: for bottling, 83–85; for brewing, 65–68; for extract, 102
Switzerland, 17
Szent-Gyorgyi, Albert, 42

Tangy kombucha marinade, 97
Tannin (tannic acid), 53–54
Tartaric acid, 29
Taste, 5, 42, 82, 88–89, 92–94
Tea, 8, 75–76, 114–16; black, 23, 70, 109, 114–15; green, 70, 109, 114–15; herbal, 109, 115–16; oolong, 70, 115; pH level, 111–14
Tea kvass, 11–12
Teepilz, 15
Temperature for brewing, 68
Teyi saki, 14
Theezwam komboecha, 15
Thiamin, 48
Threonine, 28, 41–42
Toxins, 117–18
Tryptophan, 41
Tyrosine, 28

Ultraviolet (UV) light, 68
U.S.D.A. Food Pyramid, 106
United States, 18
Urine color, 37
Uses for kombucha, 91–104, 116
Usnic acid, 30

Valine, 28, 41–42
Vinegar, 5
Vitamin B_1, 27, 48
Vitamin B_2, 27, 48
Vitamin B_3, 27, 48
Vitamin B_5, 27, 48
Vitamin B_6, 27, 48–49
Vitamin B_{12}, 27, 49
Vitamin B_{15}, 27, 49
Vitamin C, 25, 27, 32–33, 42–47
Vitamin D, 53

Water, 70
Water retention, 34, 41
Weight loss, 34
White sugar. *See* Sugar
White warts, on top of culture, 110

Yeast, 3–4, 39–40; allergies, 117; components, 40–53; reproduction, 3–4
Yin Yang Harmony Drink, 59

KOMBUCHA BREWING INSTRUCTIONS

If you decide to give away the offsprings of your kombucha culture, always be sure to also include a complete set of instructions for brewing the tea. I've heard too many comments from people who simply received a slimy thing in a bag from a friend and were left to figure out what to do with it. If you care enough to give someone a kombucha, take the extra step to ensure that they'll continue the brewing tradition safely.

I also recommend that you post a copy of instructions in your kitchen, for quick reference. Having a "cheat sheet" near your brewing area will help you to keep from missing any steps of the brewing process.

SUPPLIES FOR BREWING KOMBUCHA TEA

Avoid supplies that contain metals other than stainless steel, such as aluminum. If you use glazed ceramic containers, be sure the glazing doesn't contain lead, which can leach into the brew. Clear glass (not leaded crystal) containers are generally your safest bet.

- 4-quart glass, stainless steel or enameled pot
- Glass measuring cup
- Wooden spoons
- Large 4-quart glass container

- 1 tightly woven cotton cloth
- Tape (optional)
- Fastener for the cloth, such as rubber bands or twine
- A warm, quiet, dark, well-ventilated place

INGREDIENTS

The ingredients for kombucha brewing are simple and, except for the kombucha culture and its "starter" liquid, easy to purchase at any market.

- 2–5 black tea bags
- 3 quarts of distilled or filtered water
- 1 cup (8 ounces) white sugar (using honey or any type of sugar other than white can contaminate the culture)

- 1 kombucha culture
- ½ cup "starter" liquid (brew from the previous batch) or cider vinegar or combination of the two

Ten Steps to Brewing Success

Post these instructions where you'll be sure to review them each time you make a new batch of kombucha brew.

1. Start with a clean kitchen: free of dirt, dirty objects, fresh fruit or houseplants. Keep your hands clean throughout this process, too.

2. Bring three quarts of water to a boil. As it is heating up, stir in 1 cup of white sugar.

3. Just after the water comes to a boil, turn off the stove and remove the pot from the burner. Add 2–5 tea bags. (The more tea bags you use the stronger the tea will be.)

4. Let the tea steep for 10 minutes, then remove the tea bags.

5. Let the tea cool down until it is between lukewarm and room temperature.

6. Pour the tea into the fermentation bowl. Add the ½ cup of unfiltered "starter" liquid.

7. Place the kombucha culture on top of the tea, shiny side up, rougher side down.

8. If you're using a container with a very wide mouth, cover the top of the fermentation container with strips of tape.

9. Cover the fermentation container with a cloth. Secure it.

10. Place the fermentation container in your "kombucha brewing spot." Leave it in this spot for 5–10 days. (The longer it stays, the tarter the brew will taste.)

Bottling the Results

Make sure all your supplies are squeaky clean and your kitchen is free of potential contaminants. You will need the following supplies:

- One large plate
- Glass storage containers with tops
- Cheescloth or loosely woven cotton fabric
- Plastic funnel

1. Carefully remove the fermentation container from the kombucha brewing spot. Take off the cloth and tape.

2. Remove the cultures (yes, there's a new one there—probably on top of the "mother") from the brew and place them on a clean plate.

3. Pour the brew through the cheesecloth and funnel it into your containers.

4. Cap the bottles and store in the refrigerator.

5. Get started on the next batch of kombucha beverage and then enjoy drinking the beverage.

Drinking the Kombucha Beverage

How much of this beverage should you drink? Start off slowly—probably with about 2 ounces (¼ cup) per day. Gradually increase the amount you drink to 4 ounces (½ cup) per day. Most folks recommend drinking the tea in the morning before you eat breakfast. Drink no more than three 4-ounce glasses (1½ cups) of kombucha beverage per day.

SPECIAL NOTE: Brewing and drinking the kombucha beverage can be a healthful experience if you follow the instructions carefully and never take shortcuts. This sheet summarizes the instructions. If you have a medical condition, especially one that weakens your immune system (such as diabetes or HIV), talk to your health care provider before drinking the kombucha beverage. For more detailed instructions and information about the kombucha culture, see The Book of Kombucha *published by Ulysses Press. To order call 800-377-2542. The cost is $11.95 and shipping is free.*

ULYSSES PRESS HEALTH BOOKS

AFTER THE DIAGNOSIS
Joann LeMaistre, Ph.D.

> With the diagnosis of a chronic illness comes a blow to the psyche that can be as devastating as the symptoms. This book, written by a psychologist who has multiple sclerosis, explains how chronically ill people can be able-hearted when it is no longer possible to be able-bound. $12.95

BREAKING THE AGE BARRIER: STAYING YOUNG, HEALTHY AND VIBRANT
Helen Franks

> Drawing on the latest medical research, *Breaking the Age Barrier* explains how the proper lifestyle can stop the aging process and make you feel youthful and vital. $12.95

COUNT OUT CHOLESTEROL
Art Ulene, M.D. and Val Ulene, M.D.

> Complete with counter and detailed dietary plan, this companion resource to the *Count Out Cholesterol Cookbook* shows how to design a cholesterol-lowering program that's right for you. $12.95
> *Count Out Cholesterol Cookbook*, $14.95

IRRITABLE BOWEL SYNDROME: A NATURAL APPROACH
Rosemary Nicol

> This book offers a natural approach to a problem millions of sufferers have. The author clearly defines the symptoms and offers a dietary and stress-reduction program for relieving the effects of this disease. $9.95

KNOW YOUR BODY: THE ATLAS OF ANATOMY
Introduction by Trevor Weston, M.D.

> Designed to provide a comprehensive and concise guide to the structure of the human body, *Know Your Body* offers more than 250 color illustrations. An easy-to-follow road map of the human body. $12.95

LAST WISHES: A HANDBOOK TO GUIDE YOUR SURVIVORS
Lucinda Page Knox, M.S.W. and Michael D. Knox, Ph.D.

> A simple do-it-yourself workbook, *Last Wishes* helps people put their affairs in order and eases the burden on survivors. It allows them to plan their own funeral and leave final instructions for survivors. $12.95

LOSE WEIGHT WITH DR. ART ULENE
Art Ulene, M.D.

> This best-selling weight-loss book offers a 28-day program for taking off the pounds and keeping them off forever. $12.95

MOOD FOODS
Dr. William Vayda

> *Mood Foods* shows how the foods you eat can influence your emotions, behavior and personality. It also explains how a proper diet can help to alleviate such common complaints as PMS, hyperactivity, mood swings and stress. $9.95

PANIC ATTACKS: A NATURAL APPROACH
Shirley Trickett

> Addresses the problem of panic attacks using a holistic approach. Focusing on diet and relaxation, the book helps you prevent future attacks. $8.95

SECRETS OF SEXUAL BODY LANGUAGE
Martin Lloyd-Elliott

> This book unlocks the secret messages and sexual implications of body language. It shows how to use nonverbal communication to understand the sexual intentions of others and to send messages that properly convey one's true feelings. $16.95

THE VITAMIN STRATEGY
Art Ulene, M.D. and Val Ulene, M.D.

> A game plan for good health, this book helps readers design a vitamin and mineral program tailored to their individual needs. $11.95

YOUR NATURAL PREGNANCY: A GUIDE TO COMPLEMENTARY THERAPIES
Anne Charlish

> This timely book brings together the many complementary therapies such as aromatherapy, massage, homeopathy, acupressure, herbal medicine and meditation, that can benefit pregnant women. $16.95

To order these or other Ulysses Press books call 800-377-2542 or write to Ulysses Press, P.O. Box 3440, Berkeley, CA 94703-3440. All retail orders are shipped free of charge. California residents must include sales tax. Allow two to three weeks for delivery.

ABOUT THE AUTHOR & ILLUSTRATOR

Beth Ann Petro, M.A. is an award-winning writer, editor and instructional designer of health and safety educational publications and videos. Her more than 100 publications have been read or viewed by well over a million people, ranging from the general public to health professionals. She has taken an active, personal interest in health food trends since 1977. When not busy writing, she and her husband tend their orchard and garden at their hillside home overlooking Watsonville in California's Pajaro Valley.

Born in England, Robert Holmes launched his U.S. photography career in 1976 when Ansel Adams asked him to come work in the United States. His photographs have appeared in most of the major travel magazines including *National Geographic*, *Geo*, *Islands* and *Travel & Leisure*. In addition to his magazine credits, he has 18 books in print including The Thomas Cook Guides to California, Boston & New England, and Hawaii, as well as Fodor's *Essential California*. He lives in Mill Valley, California, with his wife and two daughters.